P9-CJF-656

Preface

The transition from university to industry could be challenging for many young professionals. This was the case with us as well. Despite a fair understanding of pharmacology and drug development, we felt the lack of operational knowledge while planning and managing a clinical trial in the first years of our career in the industry. Through this present book, we strive to bridge this gap.

This book has been written for life science graduates aspiring to work in clinical research industry or clinical research professionals without considerable experience in trial operation. It would also be useful for professionals with focused responsibilities to broaden understanding of the entire gamut of trial operation. As fundamental approach is independent of nature of the investigational product (e.g. drug, device, vaccine or diagnostic agent), we are hopeful of its wider usefulness to the entire healthcare industry.

The objective is to provide a broad outline of key activities, principles, roles, and responsibilities without getting into procedural details. Most organizations involved in clinical research have defined processes and procedures to carry out specific responsibilities relevant to their business. Hence, the discussion is purposefully limited to an overview to keep it concise yet informative. Discussion in each topic covers the background, operational overview, and usual challenges.

Frequently used terminology has been introduced in the context of specific topics to induce familiarity. The book has been organized into several topics from the perspective of a project manager driving an entire trial. Organization of topics is according to the flow of trial operation from conception to the end. At the outset, the context of different trials according to phases of drug development has been introduced. Subsequent topics are on planning, setup, execution, and closeout in a sequential manner. Towards the end, the topics are on few general aspects of trial operation.

1

This book has been written based on our practical experience, as well as regulatory guidance and other freely accessible literature. Good clinical practice (GCP) lays down the fundamental guiding principles for trial operation. Familiarity with any GCP guidance is highly recommended for best outcome from this book.

In this second edition, besides routine changes, we have added several new topics of interest.

We look forward to hearing from you. Kindly send your feedback or suggestion to *trialoperation@gmail.com*.

About the authors

Shibadas Biswal, MBBS, MD

Shibadas is a medical doctor with residency training in pharmacology from PGIMER, Chandigarh, India. He is working in the pharmaceutical industry in the field of clinical research since 2006.

Vinu M Jose, MBBS, MD, DM

Vinu is a medical doctor with residency training in pharmacology from CMC, Vellore, India, and further residency training in clinical pharmacology from PGIMER, Chandigarh, India. He is working in the pharmaceutical industry in the field of clinical research since 2007. In the past, he has held a faculty position in pharmacology.

The authors bring over 25 years of collective experience in planning and conducting clinical trials in the academic setting and pharmaceutical industry for development of generics, new chemical entities, biologics, biosimilars, vaccines, and devices.

Disclosure: The book is based on our understanding and opinion in the field, and does not in any manner reflect the opinion of any of our present or past employer. We have tried to provide factually correct information and regret any inadvertent inaccuracy. We would appreciate your kindness to bring an error to our attention at *trialoperation@gmail.com*.

Contents

1. Introduction

Healthcare interventions are essential for diagnosis, prevention, or cure of diseases, and are indispensable to the practice of modern medicine. These may be drugs, devices, vaccines, or diagnostic products. Irrespective of the intervention, the clinical development process is broadly similar with minor variations; however, it is complex, time-consuming and resource intensive. Clinical trials are human experimentation to demonstrate safety and efficacy of investigational products in a controlled manner before market authorization.

Drug discovery and development is an incremental scientific knowledge gathering process. A significant understanding of a potential drug comes from basic research, which includes target identification and preclinical evaluation of pharmacological effects. The clinical development comprises of gradual investigation in clinical pharmacology, therapeutic exploratory, and therapeutic confirmatory trials. After thorough investigation and establishment of safety/efficacy, market authorization is granted. Further investigations are continued in therapeutic use trials to understand other aspects, which were not evaluated earlier. In the current times, absolute serendipity is rare in drug discovery and development.

Pharmaceutical and healthcare companies are the usual sponsors of clinical trials in the industrial setting. Trials are conducted in healthy subjects or patients at hospitals and clinical pharmacology units. The scope of clinical trial operation includes complex steps of planning and execution. Major activities are protocol development, cost estimation, securing permissions to conduct the trial, site selection, trial setup, subject management, monitoring, data management, statistical analysis, and reporting. Many of these activities may be outsourced to contract research organizations depending on the business model.

While clinical trials are imperative for progress in medical knowledge, it can be inherently risky from the outset. It is conducted in a highly regulated environment considering the ethical and legal issues surrounding human experimentation. Thus, trial subject management is significantly different from routine patient care. Moreover, many of these experiments are conducted in healthy subjects or patients who do not get any direct or guaranteed medical benefit from it.

In this backdrop, the clinical trial operation can be further complicated in today's integrated world due to the interplay of diverse cultures, regulations, authorities, organizations, and business models. It is important to appreciate that we are enjoying the benefits of medical knowledge only due to the prior participation of fellow human beings in clinical trials.

The trial subjects are the focus of attention in a clinical trial. The entire regulatory framework of trial planning and conduct has evolved to protect rights of subjects and safeguard their health. In this respect, the investigator is on the frontline, the sponsor has the ultimate responsibility, the regulatory authorities and ethics committees have a supervisory role. The motivation for trial participation is not straightforward and can be debatable; however, voluntary participation is the essence of ethical research.

The outcome of trials may have significant implications as it supports development programs for investigational products. Next set of trials may be designed, or product approvals may be granted based on trial outcomes. The operational framework ensures data quality and integrity. Standard operating procedures minimize operator dependency. Training is integrated into the operational framework for effective compliance with regulations, ethical principles, protocol, and other standard expectations.

Clinical trials could be massive projects depending on the sample size, duration, and the disease population. For instance, several countries, organizations, and personnel along with a considerable budget may be involved in a typical phase III trial. Project management principles are applied in planning and execution to stay within defined timelines and budget to deliver credible trial data. Management of stakeholders, budget, timeline, risk, deviations, and quality is essential for effective clinical trial operation.

2. Clinical trials or human research in drug development

World Health Organization defines clinical trials as any research study that prospectively assigns human participants or groups of humans to one or more health-related interventions to evaluate the effects on health outcomes. Typical interventions include new or generic drugs, biological or biosimilars products, vaccines, medical devices, psychotherapy, surgical procedures, etc. Clinical trials may also be conducted for epidemiological research and evaluation of diagnostic agents.

While the basic approach to conducting clinical trials with different interventions is similar, there is some specific uniqueness to each of them. Often the questions to be answered are decided by the data requirement for regulatory registration. The operating business scenarios of the sponsors, expected questions to be answered, trial setting, the profile of study participants, invasiveness of the interventions, and expected benefits from trial participation influence the trial operations in a big way.

The new drugs or biological products are evaluated through a well-established incremental step wise process. A series of (e.g. 15 or more) clinical trials over 10-15-year timeframe with considerable amount of budget commitment is usually needed. Initial small trials (n=50-100) in healthy subjects in well-controlled phase 1 centers are followed by evaluation in smaller trials in target patient population to show proof of concept.

Large-scale patient trials (n> 1000) later must conclusively prove safety and efficacy of the investigational products before registration. Post registration clinical trials are also necessary to answer further questions relevant to its use in routine practice. Sponsors of these clinical trials are typically big pharmaceutical or healthcare companies.

Generic drug development typically relies on a few comparative pharmacokinetic clinical trials. There is often intense competition to reach the market after patent expiry with minimal flexibility in terms of timelines. Such trials are often conducted in healthy adult subjects in phase 1 centers with access to well-trained manpower, resources, laboratory, and a readily available pool of healthy volunteers. It is not unusual to find centres with the capability to house 50- 200 subjects and running multiple trials at a time. While such trials are simpler due to high experience of such centres or sponsors conducting similar trials, high degree of regulatory scrutiny is the norm. Typically, time available to complete the clinical development phase is few months to a couple of years.

Clinical trials settings for vaccine development range from well-resourced phase 1 centers for early phase investigation to resource-limited settings in developing countries for late phase trials. Target population for novel vaccine investigation is often pediatric population. It is not unusual to have clinical sites managing over thousand subjects in remote locations in late phase efficacy trials. Longer regulatory or ethics committee approval times, ethical challenges, significant training needs, logistics issues, need to create infrastructure at new sites, and potential for media attention are usual.

Biosimilars, the generic variant for biological molecules, need limited range of clinical development programs with comparative PK/PD and safety/efficacy trials showing similarity with the approved reference product. The clinical programs are complex in comparison to generic small molecule development and need higher budget and timeline (3-5 years) commitment. Operationally, the challenges are recruiting patients from the target population who have access to approved products and getting the necessary interest from investigators who perceive lack of any scientific novelty in comparison to trials involving newer investigational products.

Medical devices involve a diverse group of products with different utilities. Clinical development typically consists of first pilot trials in 10-30 patients followed by pivotal trials in 150-300 patients with a focus on safety. Long-term data requirement in the post-approval phase is like drugs or vaccines. These trials are not conducted in healthy subjects and are not typically blinded, randomized, or controlled. Specific skill sets of physicians, technicians or patients are needed for use of devices with a learning curve. Operationally finding trained clinical sites and willing patients depending on invasiveness of the procedures as well as training are key considerations.

Epidemiological studies evaluate patterns and causes of diseases or outcome of diseases, interventions, or other agents. These are typically conducted by academic or organization involved in public health. In the industry setting vaccine companies may conduct such investigations. In case-control studies, subjects are enrolled based on their disease status to find causes retrospectively, while in cohort studies subjects are enrolled based on their exposure status to prospectively follow for disease occurrence in comparison to controls. Operationally, epidemiological studies are large projects with considerable interaction with public institutions, community involvement and logistical challenges.

3. Clinical development plan

Clinical development plan (CDP) is a document detailing the strategy for the development of a pharmaceutical candidate through clinical phases of development. It provides a roadmap to achieve the targeted product profile (TPP) i.e. the intended characteristics, features and competitive advantage of a pharmaceutical candidate under development. Individual clinical trials are small steps of the usually complex drug development programs that contribute to the overall clinical development of a product.

A clinical development plan outlines individual trials taking into consideration the unmet medical need, potential therapeutic indications, speculated product characteristics, risk-benefit profile, key markets, regulatory strategy for market access, important milestones, criteria for decision making after each milestone, developmental costs, risks and challenges in development and competitors. It elaborates the concept of each trial and its contribution to the TPP. Individual trials assess certain characteristics of the investigational product such as safety, tolerability, proof of mechanism, pharmacokinetics, efficacy, etc.

The CDP may be limited to early phase development when the full development strategy is not clear. It may also cover important questions about the product that would be evaluated after marketing authorization e.g. long-term efficacy, safety, or health economics, etc. It is a live document and is periodically updated with the availability of new preclinical and clinical data during product development consistent with the TPP. The regulatory and commercial strategy of the product may significantly influence the CDP beyond scientific rationale.

Pediatric Study Plan (PSP) in the United States and Paediatric Investigational Plan (PIP) in the European Union are needed as per regulations to perform studies in the pediatric population to support the use of medicines in children. PSP and PIP are mandatory unless waived (i.e. not needed) or deferred (i.e.

deferred to the post-marketing stage). This requirement has evolved to mitigate paucity of information on safe use of pharmaceutical products in children; in return, pharmaceutical companies are rewarded with certain incentives.

Organizations may also have specific development plans for regional or country-specific needs depending on business strategy. For example, ethnic sensitivity study may be needed for registration in certain countries. A certain amount of local clinical data may be needed for registration in certain countries. Typically, the CDP would cover all these requirements.

From an operational standpoint, it is important to understand each trial in the perspective of the clinical development plan. The context of the trial, timelines, dependencies, importance, and country preference can be easily understood when viewed in the light of CDP.

4. Concept of the safety database and integrated analysis

The safety database refers to the number of subjects and duration of exposure to the investigational product (specifically target population) in a drug development program especially at the time of marketing authorization application. Adequate size of the safety database is an important consideration while planning a range of trials at a program level. It is not straight forward and depends on several factors such as novelty, availability of alternate therapies, target population, disease condition, duration of intended use and any safety signals from preclinical and early phase trials.

This is a usual topic of discussion with regulatory authorities early in the product development and an important consideration for planning clinical trials while choosing sample size, clinical trial population and minimum enrolment at country level in phase 3 trials.

Integrated analysis of safety and efficacy in pooled datasets from multiple clinical trials is performed to support marketing authorization application. The aim is to assess the overall evidence for efficacy, any rare adverse events or safety signals in a larger sample size and any variability of safety or efficacy in different subgroups (e.g. old age, subjects with diabetes). Subtle differences exist between data integration and pooling and are outside the scope of this discussion.

Several complexities are involved in integrated data analysis and summary report preparation. The usual issues are defining regulatory expectations, the structure of an integrated database, clinical considerations, datasets from trials to be pooled, defining subgroups, managing differences in the structure of individual trial datasets and prompt availability of trial data. Like individual studies, a statistical analysis plan is developed to govern the integrated analysis with details of the approaches, methods, and format of statistical outputs. It is a multi-functional endeavor managed by a team with representatives from clinical, regulatory, statistics, programming, pharmacovigilance, and medical writing groups.

While this topic may not be directly relevant from a clinical trial operation perspective, it is an important consideration while planning individual trials. The similarity in assessment and visit structures, common trial databases and data standards for individual trials make it easier for later integrated analysis.

5. Developing study designs or concepts for a program

Fundamentally, clinical trials in drug development programs support the intended target product profile. Clinical development plans describe broadly the study concepts or designs. Often an informal study concept sheet is developed for preliminary discussion with internal and external stakeholders. Typically, feedback on feasibility, timeline and resource requirement is taken from all stakeholders including clinical operation group. The study concept sheet is often used for internal approvals; then, it becomes the basis to elaborate a protocol.

There is no established approach to design studies. However, a methodical approach helps to avoid factors that would be otherwise overlooked. Often, there is a compulsion to design studies expeditiously for several reasons. Initiating the process early provides an opportunity to think over it, consult with relevant people, and brainstorm on various aspects over time.

The clinical development process answers many questions and explores some hypotheses. These are necessary to assess the investigational product to characterize its profile as per the TPP. A good starting point is writing down questions to be answered in the clinical development program in the order of priority. While the primary questions are obvious, there are opportunities for supplementary questions that can be answered in individual clinical trials that need meticulous planning.

Attempts are made to refine and prioritize questions. Some questions need to be answered with statistical power for regulatory purposes while others need only scientific exploration. Answering multiple related questions within one study is helpful in terms of resource optimization and data comparability. General approaches are the addition of multiple evaluations, arms, or parts to a study to address multiple endpoints. Another approach is to have subsets of the study population to evaluate aspects besides the core study goals. Typically, a lean study can deliver quicker result and is preferred when that is essential.

While developing designs for individual studies, there could be more than one approach for each study. Potential designs with its pros and cons in term of its ability to answer clinical questions, strength/weakness, feasibility, and resource needs are compared to select the suitable design. Various functions are consulted for feedback on the different approaches; peer review by colleagues or external consultants are helpful. It is a good practice to note down all the questions raised, and clarifications provided. Blind copy of designs from another similar program should be avoided.

6. Managing clinical trials of several clinical development programs

A clinical development program along with its set of clinical trials is heavily dependent on the nature of the investigational product. New molecules, biologics or vaccines development need an extensive range of trials over a prolonged period while generics, biosimilars or vaccines with established correlates of protection need fewer trials over shorter periods for registration. Sponsors would typically support fewer programs with extensive development requirements, however, can support number of programs with fewer trial requirements.

The operational planning for individual programs can widely vary based on factors such as nature of the product, target country of registration, regulatory requirement, business model, development time and cost, competitive landscape, the likelihood of success and organizational priority. The complexity of the team structure and individual responsibilities can vary accordingly. For instance, individuals might be supporting one or only a few programs in case of innovative products while it could be several programs for generic or biosimilar products with lesser complexities.

Innovative product developments typically involve elaborate and comprehensive development plans, bigger teams with wider functional representation, longer development cycles, higher budgetary allocation, considerable attention to detail and frequent regulatory or external consultations. Changes and adjustments to the development plans are common. Irrespective of the nature of the products, there is a general tendency in the sponsor organizations to manage strategic elements internally while outsourcing operational elements. Adequate supervision and quality assurance measures are devised for the quality of externally supported work.

Operational and resource planning is indispensable for efficient and workable clinical development plans. Operational planning for the range of clinical trials to support development programs is built to suit specific requirements and business model of a sponsor organization. It takes into consideration available internal resources, experience, budgetary allocations, priorities, dependency on external partners and potential for changes in strategy.

Resources in terms of manpower, budget, and expertise are mapped to meet individual program requirements on a yearly basis for next 3-5 years. Each program and each trial in each program is tracked for its budget, timelines, dependencies, risks, critical issues, and key metrics.

While managing clinical trials for several programs, changes are inevitable for several reasons. Programs are prioritized due to promising results or may be terminated or reprioritized. Budgetary restrictions may lead to non-critical trials pushed to later years. On the other hand, the budget may be available as some other programs are terminated or suspended, hence, some of the trials could be advanced.

Interdependencies among trials, regulatory feedbacks, safety signal with a product, and changing competitive landscape typically affect trials in a program. Mergers, acquisitions and changing business models of R&D organizations (e.g. decision to outsource less priority work) bring in a separate set of dynamics. It is a general expectation to manage such changes efficiently with agility.

Managing peaks and troughs of workload along with product pipeline and development cycles is a significant consideration in development operations, and outsourcing is a common strategy to manage such fluctuations. Increasingly, operation leaders are part of global program teams to align with changing dynamics.

7. Responsibility within a clinical operation department

Within the broader clinical development group, the clinical operation function has evolved as a sophisticated group with various sub-functions to manage a wide range of responsibilities. Between organizations, structures may vary with similarities or differences depending on the unique set of conditions. The structure could be significantly influenced by the level of dependence on outsourcing. The structure of contract research organizations may also vary depending on the business model and areas of expertise.

Monitoring and site management are the core functions of a clinical operation organization. Field monitors, remote monitors, and their managers serve as the sponsor's representatives to oversee study conduct as per the protocol and regulations; all communications between the sponsor and clinical sites are routed through them. There are also the functions, which are outsourced to external partners.

Typically, each trial is managed by a project manager who coordinates with other functions to ensure that the trial is executed as per the protocol with acceptable quality. Compliance with regulations, budget allocations, and defined timelines are basic expectations. Lead project managers oversee the work of project managers of different trials in a development program and manage coordination with the global program team or senior management.

Medical monitoring could be part of clinical operations function to provide scientific support to the clinical trial team and investigators (e.g. clarifications on the protocol, investigational product, AE management, clinical data review, etc). Medical monitors maintain scientific relationships with important investigators and manage trial related external communications.

The clinical trial operation is a process intensive function to comply with regulations and ensure quality. Process management group has a vital role to ensure availability of necessary and streamlined processes in the form of SOPs, work practices as well as its periodic updates and implementation. It may also work with the quality assurance group to coordinate audits/inspections as well as the implementation of corrective and preventive actions (CAPAs) as a part of the quality management system (QMS).

Training coordinators are responsible for designing strategies for delivery of various training modules, SOPs as well as tracking training compliance. This function may be part of process management group.

Numerous documents are produced during clinical trials that need to be collected, quality checked and organized in the trial master file (paper or electronic). Various dossiers are prepared for regulatory or ethic committee submissions and the documents must be readily available at the time of audits and inspections. While some of these could be managed by the trial project managers, specialized trial document management groups are necessary for larger trials. A medical writing group may support various document drafting as well as coordination of review and finalization.

Several electronic systems are in use to support clinical trial operations such as Clinical Trial Management System (CTMS), contract and invoice management systems, electronic TMF, data visualization tools, etc. Administrators of such systems work as the primary contacts or subject matter experts for users and stakeholders. Key responsibilities include design and evaluation of processes as well as system enhancements and standards to improve clinical trial management. Other responsibilities are the creation of SOPs, system-specific documentation, training materials, and content to ensure the understanding of system users.

With outsourcing an increasingly predominant operating business model for sponsor organizations, several sub-functions have evolved to support it. Some of the responsibilities are vendor identification, evaluation, and liaison as well as management of contracts and invoices. In the vendor organizations, business development function liaisons with sponsor organizations. Complementary functions in both sponsor and vendor organizations are there to prepare and assess budget and resource requirement, oversee the progress of outsourced activities as well as conflict resolution.

8. Single and multiple ascending dose trials

These are the first studies with a compound to evaluate safety for human use and the tolerated dose range. The primary objective is to assess safety and tolerability. Pharmacokinetics of the drug is also typically evaluated (e.g. bioavailability, food effect, different routes of administration) and pharmacodynamics may be evaluated when possible depending on the mechanism of action, the population in the study and other factors (e.g. receptor binding information, the effect on an enzyme activity, other specific information).

A group of subjects is dosed with a calculated presumptive safe starting dose of the drug. This dose is derived from in vitro, preclinical and simulation studies. Regulatory authorities have put forth guidance on how to calculate a safe starting dose. If the dose is found safe, another group of subjects is dosed with the next higher dose level. Incremental dose levels are administered until study stopping rule is reached and the maximal tolerated dose is decided. In a single ascending dose (SAD) study, only a single dose (just one time) is administered, while in a multiple ascending dose (MAD) study, repeated doses (e.g. once daily for 5 days) are administered to each group of the subjects at each dose level. The intention of administering multiple doses is to reach steady-state conditions when drug intake and clearance from the body have stabilized.

Usually, the studies are conducted in healthy subjects except in specific situations, where drugs may be too toxic for healthy subjects (e.g. in the setting of cancer drugs). There could be other scientific reasons for a change from the standard approach. For instance, a drug with hypotensive properties may be better tolerated in patients with hypertension if the drug is under development for such an indication. When there are such considerations, subjects who are otherwise healthy or have specific derangement may be the suitable population of a trial. There could be a multistage approach as well, with initial evaluation in healthy subjects and subsequent evaluation in the target population.

It is essential to have domiciled environment for close monitoring and multiple intensive assessments. The study plan is driven by pharmacology of the compound, its perceived or predicted effects and nature of potential adverse events. Staggered enrolment (e.g. 2 subjects from a group of 8 are dosed followed by a period of observation for safety, then dosing of another 2 subjects and so on) at each dose level could be used to minimize the overall risk to the subjects. Placebo control, randomization, and blinding are usual features to prevent bias and correctly attribute adverse events to the investigational products. Confounding factors are minimized by enforcing a controlled environment. However, depending on specific scenarios, various approaches or modifications can be employed.

The protocol needs to be flexible in terms of study drug dose modifications based on safety or pharmacokinetic data without the need to go back to the ethics committee and health authority for approval. A safety monitoring committee, sponsor's medical expert and the investigator may jointly take this decision based on the available data from the earlier dose levels. For instance, a dose level may be repeated, or a dose escalation may be less than the planned next dose level based on the emerging safety and pharmacokinetics data. It could be especially important for a new class of compounds as the observed effects may be significantly different from the predicted effects.

Operationally, these are simple studies and are conducted in well-equipped clinical pharmacology units (phase 1 centers). There may be issues with approval from health authorities and some countries are more open to such studies. Due to the flexibility expected, the clinical site may be selected in a country with the favorable regulatory environment and with faster ethics committee review timelines. A well-equipped and well-experienced center (with an experienced investigator) is also favored by both sponsors and health authorities.

Constant evaluation of the safety data is integral to first in man studies and frequent meetings between the sponsor and the investigators are usually needed during study conduct. Arrangements for quick pharmacokinetic evaluation to take decisions on the maximum dose level (to be evaluated) are typically needed. Recruitment is typically not an issue with healthy subject studies, while it could be problematic when looking for specific patient populations.

9. Pharmacokinetics trial

Bioavailability, bioequivalence, food effect, drug-drug interaction, pharmacokinetics (PK) in special population or specific disease states and ethnic sensitivity studies are included in this group where the primary objective is an estimation of PK parameters. In simple terms, PK is about measuring levels of drugs or metabolites in biological fluids (e.g. blood, urine, CSF, peritoneal fluid, milk, semen, etc) and calculating its parameters. The PK parameters are a set of values to indicate how the physiological system handles a drug. The most important PK parameters are Cmax (highest level of drug achieved), AUC (area under the curve of drug levels at different time points) and Tmax (time of Cmax).

Bioavailability can be defined as the degree to which or the rate at which a drug or other substance is absorbed or becomes available at the site of physiological activity. In a bioequivalence study, bioavailability from two different formulations or route of administrations is compared. In a food effect study, the effect of diet on bioavailability is evaluated to recommend on drug intake in relation to food. Drug-drug interaction studies evaluate the potential effect of a drug on the PK of another drug; the mechanism of interactions could be interference with absorption, distribution, metabolism, excretion, or protein binding. Such studies are thus essential for a recommendation on co-prescription of other drugs. The PK of drugs may be altered in specific disease states (e.g. hepatic failure, renal failure) or populations (e.g. pediatric, geriatric, gender effects, ethnic backgrounds) which may warrant dose modification; hence, it is evaluated.

Variability of PK parameters is an important consideration in the design of PK studies. PK parameters may have significant intra-subject (differences in the same subject on separate occasions) and inter-subject (differences from subject to subject) variability. Inter-subject variability is typically higher than the intra-subject variability. Hence, a crossover design is preferred i.e. a group of subjects is administered study drugs on separate occasions and blood or other biological fluid of interest is collected for measurement of levels. A washout period between occasions of drug administration allows clearance of drug/metabolites from the body before the next administration. This is by far the most common and cost-effective design. At times, when variability is high, replicate design may be utilized i.e. each of the test/reference formulation is administered more than once to each subject. In the case of drugs with a long half-life, cross over design may not be operationally feasible, and a parallel design is preferred. When the effect of the disease states on PK is evaluated, the studies are conducted in subjects with the specific disease and a matched healthy control (matched for age, gender, body mass index, etc).

The basic evaluation in any PK study is a collection of biological fluid of interest at different time points to calculate PK parameters after a treatment administration. 'Treatment' refers to the different conditions for comparison. It could be different drug formulations in a bioequivalence study, drug with and without meals (or the different type of meals) in a food effect study, and drug with or without an interacting drug in a drug-drug interaction study. The duration of each occasion of treatment and subsequent sample collection is called a period. In this perspective, there may be as many periods as the number of treatments separated by washout periods (to ensure elimination of drug or its metabolites from the body). The sequence of administration of treatments is randomized to minimize the effect of any period on the treatments. Typically, PK studies are open-label because of the objectivity of the assessment and minimal effect of treatment allocation information in well-controlled trial conditions.

PK of drugs may be easily influenced by factors such as time of drug administration, food intake, concomitant medication, posture after drug intake, the volume of fluid intake, lifestyle, or smoking. Standardization of such factors is essential to minimize confounding factors. Restrictions are selected based on the known properties of the drug or as per general recommendations. Typically, PK studies are conducted in clinical pharmacology units (phase 1 centers) and subjects are domiciled to have better control of the conditions as well as to facilitate frequent sample collection. Hospital settings are preferred for PK in disease states.

Most PK studies are conducted in healthy adult subjects. However, subjects from other populations are recruited to investigate PK in disease states. Depending on the population in question, the study could be easy or difficult to recruit and conduct. For instance, conducting a PK study in pediatric population could be very challenging. Certain drugs may not be tolerated in healthy subjects e.g. psychotropic or oncology medications. Studies in post-menopausal women, renal failure or hepatic failure patients have its own unique challenges. In most cases, there is no direct benefit to the subjects in these studies. Many of the PK studies are meant for regulatory submission and hence, sensitive with respect to quality. It could be pivotal studies, which lead to marketing authorization in certain countries. Drug product and PK sample handling is typically the subject of regulatory scrutiny during an inspection.

Operational uniqueness:

- PK studies in healthy subjects are conducted in highly sophisticated controlled centers and a very high standard of quality is expected to lead to pressure situations. Centers should be selected after a thorough audit. The experience of conducting of pivotal marketing authorization studies is given importance.

- Ethical concerns always surround these studies as subjects do not get any therapeutic benefit. Regulatory timelines, cost, recruitment rate may be favourable in certain countries and centers; hence, an appropriate center needs to be selected depending on the situation.

- Specialized centers are available that have the experience to conduct studies in specific disease populations.

- PK studies in patients are typically challenging in terms of recruitment. Concomitant medications and associated diseases need to be considered in entry criteria and restrictions while conducting studies in disease states such as hepatic or renal failure.

- PK studies are commonly conducted in healthy male subjects.

- Regulatory and ethics committee concerns are usual in PK studies in frail patients or pediatric population.

10.Therapeutic exploratory trial

Drug development begins with building a biological concept or hypothesis e.g. how a drug could affect the physiological or pathological process of human body. Once safety and tolerability margins have been explored in tolerability (Phase 1) studies, the next step is the demonstration that a drug works in the target indication in patient population and thereby, proving the hypothesis. The therapeutic exploratory studies are crucial first steps to evaluate any potential benefit of manipulating a biological process. It ranges from proof of concept studies to get the first indication of efficacy to other studies (e.g. dose-ranging studies) aimed at gathering information needed to plan therapeutic confirmatory trials, which are the basis of regulatory approval. Typically, such studies come under phase II of the drug development phases. Interestingly, any further investment in a drug development program depends on the promise shown in such studies.

Here are few usual objectives of such studies:

- Exploration of safety and efficacy in target population

- Finding dose and treatment regimen for a new drug for a target population
- Evaluation of human pharmacology study results in target population
- Exploration and validation of efficacy measures

The scenarios can be widely different when planning such trials. Human experience may be limited to only tolerability data from first in man studies or extensive, in case, the drug was tested or approved in other indications. Often, it is a very exciting moment for the company and the team working on the compound. Study designs could be innovative with adaptive features to accommodate the lack of previous experience or expected magnitude of drug effect. For instance, sample size may have to be reworked or dose need to be modified in a treatment arm during the trial.

Every effort is made to minimize any confounding factors that may influence the study result such as co-morbidities, co-medications, life styles, study conduct, evaluations, and so on. Randomization, blinding and control arms (placebo/active controls) are included to maximize validity of the results. In a way, all the measures are taken as feasible to accurately demonstrate any potential efficacy of the drug. Study duration is dependent on the accepted disease measures (efficacy endpoints) to explore drug effect. Surrogate endpoints are often used in such studies. Safety monitoring is planned based on the tolerability issues identified with the drug in earlier studies, the safety profile of the drug class and disease condition under evaluation.

Such trials are typically conducted in patients. Usually, the sample size is less than a hundred, and only a few clinical sites are involved. Duration of the trials may range from few weeks to few months. Scale of trial operation can be of medium complexity between the well-controlled phase 1 trials and the close to real life scenario late phase trials. Frequency of visits, evaluations, monitoring, supervision, and strict compliance requirements make these trials very demanding for patients and investigators. Several exploratory measures are usually assessed.

These studies usually have strict stopping rules, periodic interim analysis with go/no go criteria and data review by data safety monitoring committees.

Operational uniqueness:

- Extensive safety data is not usually available while conducting these trials and may lead to concerns from health authorities. Countries with experienced health authorities may be considered for faster approval.

- Clinical sites with experience in translational medicine trials should be selected with capabilities and advanced setup as per protocol requirements. Sites should have experience with similar studies, which require intense involvement and close follow up of the subjects. The investigator and the staff should have the time and motivation for such trials. Specialized centers have come up that cater to such requirements and should be preferred.

- Increasingly, therapeutic exploratory studies are conducted to find treatments for rare and neglected diseases. Recruitment, retention, compliance issues should be discussed with the investigators upfront while planning the protocol. Strict requirements and narrow entry criteria may make such studies difficult to run compared to other patient trials.

- Specialized equipment, evaluation scales, exploratory evaluations/biomarkers, etc. are usually part of these studies. Identification of such service providers and validity of the methodology are typical concerns. Hence, study feasibility evaluation is crucial along with protocol development.

- Due to short duration or exploratory nature, patients may not get direct benefit in true sense; however, the trials could be demanding in terms of several visits and evaluations. Committed patients are also essential for these studies.

- Registration in public domain websites such as clinicalTrials.gov is essential, and there could be hesitation from the sponsor to make sensitive information public at this stage. Deliberation to publish minimum required information and scrutiny by intellectual property attorneys are common.

11.Therapeutic confirmatory trial

Therapeutic confirmatory studies are conducted with the intention to obtain regulatory approval for marketing authorization in the target countries. Hence, study design, endpoints, duration, comparative drug, entry criteria, sample size and statistical analysis need to be identified in the protocol as per the available regulatory guidance. Direct discussions with the concerned regulatory authorities are often conducted for this early in the drug development program.

During drug development, human pharmacology and therapeutic exploratory studies build or explore the conceptual framework in humans that was conceived in preclinical and laboratory setting. Many of the exploratory studies also gather information to effectively conduct a therapeutic confirmatory trial. Efficacy may be evaluated in the exploratory studies; however, it may not have the statistical power or other strengths in terms of universally accepted disease endpoints, duration of evaluation, comparison to the standard of care or study conduct in a comparable real-life scenario.

Confirmatory trials are conducted with the objective to conclusively demonstrate therapeutic benefit and establish the safety of a new drug in the target patient population. It is usually conducted in phase III of the drug development phase and is often the last set of trials before regulatory approval is applied for marketing authorization. From a design perspective, these trials are often randomized, parallel group, controlled (placebo and standard of care), blinded and well powdered to conclusively demonstrate efficacy. The trials are designed comprehensively to assess the utility of the new drug to medical practice. Multiple dose levels of the new drug may be evaluated to show any dose-effect response. Operationally, the scale of these studies could be huge with thousands of patients in hundreds of centers in several countries running for few years involving a considerable proportion of the drug development budget. The scale may be smaller and of shorter duration in specific situations.

Endpoints of such trials are generally 'hard endpoints' which are more conclusive such as mortality, measures of disease progression, disease control over a clinically significant timeframe, incidence of complications or improvement in quality of life. In comparison, the endpoints in exploratory trials are indicative such as a change in biomarkers.

Protocol development involves a detailed consultation process for feasibility as well as data acceptability. An end of phase II consultation meeting is often the norm for guidance from health authorities on the further development of the drug, trial design or data requirements for market authorization. Similarly, the study design is also discussed with key opinion leaders for expert guidance. It ensures that the approach to proving the utility of a new drug would be acceptable to the medical community when approved for use in case of a successful trial.

The sponsors may run the trial using their own trial operation team or may choose to outsource it to one or more contract research organizations (CRO). Once a synopsis is worked out, feedback is invited from different countries on feasibility; it includes feedback from potential investigators and health authorities on study design, entry criteria and assessments. Feasibility information is also obtained on recruitment targets and timelines. Investigator selection in a country or region may take into consideration the key opinion leadership status of investigators irrespective of their actual potential to recruit patients. Key opinion leaders (KOL) may bring more credibility to the trial as well as influence other investigators to participate in the trial. In case of product approval, KOLs may also facilitate market access due to their ability to influence. Hence, it is important for sponsors to get certain KOLs to have first-hand experience with the experimental drug. One or more coordinating investigators may be selected for better study management and communication with the sponsor.

Operational uniqueness:

- Studies are operationally easier for individual subject participation as protocols are made with the intention to treat the patients in real life situation as far as possible. Intensity of the visits, evaluations (especially laboratory evaluations) are less burdensome in comparison to exploratory studies. Broadly, the patient population is less homogenous in comparison to that in exploratory trials.

- More clinical sites can run such studies than the exploratory studies; however, there could still be challenges due to higher sample size and recruitment targets.

- Entry criteria and restrictions are flexible considering the target population, co-medications, co-morbidities, safety of the compound and the potential ways in which the compound is intended to be used post approval. There may be need for country specific entry criteria.

- Individual patient management could be complex due to broad entry criteria, several flexibilities, effort to mimic real life situation, co-morbidity, and co-medication. Managing subjects with poor disease control on the standard of care or the experimental treatment may be troublesome.

- Typically, the study is conducted in multiple countries, and individual country operation team of the sponsor or CRO takes a significant role in study management such as investigator selection, monitoring, drug supply, safety monitoring, clarifying questions from the sites, so on.

- Different countries and sites have varying document requirements for regulatory and ethics committee review. The approval timelines could also be widely different. The wave of site initiations in each country is driven by the timing of approvals (health authority and ethics committees). Country and site-specific regulations and procedures need to be taken into consideration for study conduct.

- Certain countries may require specific number of enrolment for consideration of market authorization. Comparative drug product requirement may differ in different countries, often it needs to be sourced from the respective countries.

- The window of recruitment timeframe is typically wider at a global level as the duration of the trials are often longer due to larger sample size.

- There may be similar compounds from competitor companies in phase III of development who would conduct similar studies at the same clinical sites. Competition at the trial sites needs to be carefully managed.

- Investigator fees, cost of similar services and subject compensation may be quite diverse in different countries.

- Some countries tend to recruit at a much faster rate than others. However, it may have to be limited depending on the original plan of recruitment target for each country for a balance of diversity.

- Rules governing confidentiality, data sharing, investigator indemnity, posting of trial information in local public websites, etc. are a few aspects to be considered on a case to case basis.

- Typically, these are big budget trials and management of financial aspects is one key aspect. When the expenditures are planned to be spread over a few years, it is important to plan and execute in a way so that there is no extra expenditure in each year or carryover of the expenditure to the next year.

- Central laboratories and central randomization through interactive response technology are the norm in such big trials.
- These trials are sensitive from a regulatory perspective and are often inspected. Effective planning for adequate documentation and archival is essential.

- Project management, coordination and tracking the study progress among the enormous team and stakeholders who are often from various backgrounds is a challenge. Milestones are set and tracked closely with contingency measures and risk mitigation plans; study timelines are considerably driven by the plan for market access.

12. Therapeutic use trial

Therapeutic use trials are part of phase IV of drug development, and are conducted post-approval to market a drug. Such trials are driven by regulatory commitments at the time of market authorization and the desire to establish safety and effectiveness of the new drug in real-life clinical practice. A distinction may be made when a trial is conducted with an approved product in an unapproved indication, as it would be categorized as therapeutic exploratory or confirmatory trial and not as therapeutic use category since the indication is still under investigation.

During the pre-approval period, the trials are more focused to bring the drug as quickly as possible to the market. Once the drug is available in the market for use upon prescription, there is an opportunity to conduct observational studies to gather information on pattern of use, compliance, rare adverse event (AE) profile, effectiveness, user preference, refinement on dose recommendation, cost-benefit, quality of life, possibility of use in subjects excluded in confirmatory trials (in certain circumstances), and so on. Physicians and investigators also get an opportunity to independently evaluate the drug besides the innovator company.

Comparative effectiveness trials may be conducted to see the benefits in comparison to existing therapies. In observational or non-interventional trials, subjects who are prescribed the drug as per routine practice are followed up systematically using an observational protocol for a period commensurate with the objective to monitor acute or chronic AEs, effectiveness, compliance, or long-term issues. Specific patients on an intervention may be enrolled into a registry for a closer follow up; it is often to answer questions limited to a subpopulation taking a drug. Trials may aim at endpoints such as quality of life, long-term mortality or morbidity and cost-effectiveness of the therapies which are of greater relevance to patients. Retrospective studies such as case-control studies are typically planned after a drug is in the market for sufficient duration. Identification of users/non-users of the drug in the population is essential for such studies.

The pattern of marketing, prescription, and use in the various clinical, social, economic scenarios can be evaluated in drug utilization studies to understand the influence of such factors or outcomes. In general, the objective of these studies is far away from the conventional safety or efficacy trials and towards a broader and in-depth understanding of the drug use in routine medical practice.

Operational uniqueness:

- Study designs are often simple focusing more on data collection in the setting of routine medical practice. The trials could have randomization, blinding or multiple arms depending on the objective. Certain studies could be similar to confirmatory trials while other may be simpler.

- Operationally, these trials are site and subject friendly with broad entry criteria and without a need for frequent visits, laboratory tests or restrictions as in routine patient care. Many sites and investigators can run such trials.

- Many of the trials are planned and driven locally at the country level taking inputs from internal medical affairs and marketing teams besides local key opinion leaders. It is usual to have commercial team suggesting potential investigators in such trials.

- For non-interventional trials, informed consent is still required for only the observational and data collection aspect. Consent may not be required for the treatment part as it is often a prerequisite to participate in the study. If any evaluations are conducted in the study that is not part of routine care, informed consent must be obtained for it as well.

- Non-interventional trials are often wrongly perceived by the investigators as means to increase sales unless it has a clear objective to answer a meaningful question.

13. Trial in special or specific population

In the current approach to drug development, specific categories of the population are excluded from the initial set of clinical trials, as treatment effect is perceived to be different. Such an approach is adopted for strategic reasons considering concerns about safety, efficacy, data variability, ethics, feasibility, and necessity. However, trials could be conducted separately for the regulatory requirement or to broaden the population where the drug can be used.

Special or specific populations are referred to people with specific illnesses (hepatic or renal failure) or subpopulations (pediatric, geriatric, specific genotypes, ethnicity, patients using specific drugs or devices, etc). The aim of such trials is to evaluate any potential difference in drug effect in such subpopulations. Not every aspect of the drug effect in these specific populations is evaluated; rather, it estimates the most important difference to understand the implications and thus, could become the basis for dose adjustment, cautionary guidance, or risk-benefit assessment.

For instance, in many situations, the pharmacokinetics (PK) of the drugs are altered and it is the basis for increased pharmacological action leading to adverse events. Patients with cardiac failure may be more sensitive to the negative inotropic effect of a drug. Geriatric patients are likely to be more sensitive to drugs with the negative effect on cognitive function. Pediatric patients need different doses or dosing regimens.

Operational uniqueness:

- Operationally, these are small trials with few subjects except in specific situations such as a confirmatory trial in a pediatric age group; however, the study conduct may not be easy due to practical challenges.

- Ethical and safety concerns may arise from ethics committees, health authorities and investigators, especially in situations where there is no direct benefit to the participating subjects (For instance, a PK study in end stage renal failure undergoing dialysis would not benefit trial subjects).

- Informed consent procedures are different in pediatric trials; assent is taken from the pediatric subjects, while consent is taken from the parents or legal guardians. The language should be much simpler to take assent from children.

- Entry criteria, restrictions and study procedures should consider practical aspects such as coexisting illnesses, intensity of sickness, feasibility, concomitant medications, and so on. Detailed background knowledge about the disease, lifestyle of these subjects and inputs of the investigators into the protocol is helpful. The investigators could review the study plan with few subjects for feedback.

- Frequent blood or other biological sample collection that requires an invasive procedure is a sensitive issue in children and frail subjects. A reasonable balance between operational feasibility and scientific requirement is crucial for success.

- Specialized centers performing trials in special population could be advantageous due to essential expertise and experience.

- Running such trials may be expensive in general when per patient cost is considered, and recruitment is typically slow.

14. Project assignment

Clinical trials run like projects and many features are indistinguishable from a conventional project such as building a road. Typically, project managers are assigned at the sponsor, service provider (contract research organization) and clinical site level to drive the trial work at respective organizations. Depending upon the workload and nature of work, project managers may handle one or several projects. Background knowledge of the project is useful to understand the expectations, deliverable and challenges involved. Not all projects have similar deliverable, attention, and enthusiasm, yet all expected to be completed in time with high quality.

Trials can vary in complexity, scale, and difficulty from an operational perspective. Important determinants include purpose, the phase of drug development, priority, team members, the investigational drug, sample size, evaluations, patient population, duration, potential countries, etc. For each team member, understanding the background is crucial to operational success. Situations can change dramatically; an otherwise simple trial may get complicated due to delay in timelines and then be in focus.

A clinical trial is conducted by a cross-functional team responsible for various aspects of trial design and conduct. The sponsor may outsource certain trial activities to other organizations depending on the business model. Thus, many of the team members may be from other organizations (service providers). It is not unusual to come across 40-50 different team members/personnel during a trial those are from within or outside the sponsor organization. Understandably, a set of people are actively involved at any given time, while others get involved at appropriate stages of the trial. Few team members are involved from start to end while the majority have responsibilities for specific activities. It is essential that team member focus on individual contribution and do not step into others' domain areas.

Clinical trials originate from the development plan or life-cycle management plan of a compound. At the sponsor level, individual trials are assigned to a project manager or an equivalent responsible person for planning and conduct. The first step is forming the trial team responsible for planning. A kick-off meeting with the key stakeholders is essential to understand the background and expectations. The core team starts drafting the protocol/synopsis from a concept sheet once the green light is obtained for a trial. A basic outline is essential for introductory discussions on the budget, outsourcing, drug supply, data management, country selection, regulatory considerations and so on.

Prior experience with a similar project is immensely valuable. A compound under development or a type of study may have a generic set of entry criteria, evaluations, regulatory constraints, or recruitment challenges. Helpful insights could be obtained through discussions with people with prior experience, review of prior trials with the same compound or similar trials with other compounds. For instance, the regulatory environment may be more favorable to conduct a trial in one country and that might be the major reason to select that country. In another situation, favorable recruitment rate could be the deciding factor. Thus, valuable time need not be wasted to find the right country.

Once a synopsis with the study outline is available as well as key expectations and issues understood, consultation with stakeholders is initiated for planning and operational feasibility. A broad understanding of the entire trial process is essential for effective planning. A broad outline of the study can be created using a project management tool for better visualization of the timelines, risks, challenges, and management expectation.

Potential major rate-limiting processes should be identified and discussed with the concerned stakeholders. The team should be aware of key issues and challenges to anticipate or take contingency measures when necessary, thus minimizing unexpected circumstances.

The timeline is a key issue and major reason for stress as trials seldom run as planned. Despite meticulous planning, most trials eventually face operational or logistic challenges at some stages. A timeline that simply considers the best-case scenario is unlikely to be achieved. Hence, practical considerations and buffer time must be considered in timeline planning to avoid unnecessary pressure. It may be prudent to discuss the best case and worst-case scenarios with the stakeholders. Quality should never be traded for timelines as nobody cares about timelines if the quality has been compromised raising a question mark on the validity of the trial outcome.

A supportive and enthusiastic team is crucial to the ultimate success and smooth progress of the trial. The team should be aligned with the priority and deliverables. For instance, if a trial result is crucial in the development stage of a compound, there is the focus from the upper management and it is natural for the team members to be attentive and accommodating. In another instance, where the trial is not in the critical path in the development, priorities of the team members may not be aligned, and it leads to lack of cooperation. Many such dynamics about a team are out of the scope of this discussion and should be understood with experience.

A complex study protocol may need multiple consultations and reviews before finalization. Similarly, a large or complex trial may involve a complex operational arrangement with multiple third parties, several clinical sites, countries, and so on. When many people get involved in a trial, the unavoidable iterative process may stretch planning and setup process. The dependency of a trial on other trial results must be considered. For instance, if the dose selection would be based on another ongoing trial, the study design cannot proceed until that result is available.

Periodic change in the plan by the management is usual and should be evaluated as and when such requests come in. Any change which may impact the timelines, cost or feasibility should be discussed with the management. Uncertainty may come from various sources, and mindfulness of such factors pays off to be prepared in case of a drastic decision of trial cancellation.

In summary, in the initial few days following the project assignment, it is highly recommended and worthwhile to spend time holding formal or informal discussions with people around to understand the background, context, issues, and priorities.

15. Project management in clinical trial

The clinical trial planning and conduct is complex due to the intricate and process intensive work. Several organizations and personnel from different background are integrated to an interdependent matrix environment. At any given time, certain tasks could be on the critical path while others are dependent on it. Each team member needs to be tuned and informed appropriately for planning and readiness for the next step. Concepts of project management are applied to the trial operation for seamless progress and to ensure everyone is aware of individual contributions, dependencies, and timelines.

The whole clinical trial work can be broken down to 'work packets' such as protocol development, study setup, clinical conduct, data management, statistics, monitoring, laboratory work and report preparations; all these are performed in an interdependent manner. These broader subdivisions also have further divisions to sub-activities. A trial manager who understands the entire process from end to end drives the project while lead team members drive individual 'work packets'.

The entire trial is charted out in a project map taking into consideration the activities, dependencies, setup time, completion time, resource requirement as well as potential scenarios which may affect operation. Milestones are laid down for the trial as well as for each activity and sub-activity, which are built into a project map. Best-case and worst-case scenario constructions help to understand practical realities of operation. The sophistication of planning depends on the complexity and the enormity of the trial.

Resource and timeline planning are critical to project management. All stakeholders should participate in planning and optimization of the plan as the trial progresses. If the entire trial or specific activities are to be performed on a priority, it must be discussed and agreed upon. Stakeholders of the trial must be identified and handled appropriately. They must be updated on the progress, consulted, and taken into confidence in decision making.

Points of contact for the whole trial and the constituent activities are identified for ease of communication and accountability. The study manager is responsible for the overall study conduct in time, within budget and with quality as well as coordination with the trial team and other stakeholders (e.g. management). Similarly, there could be leads for each major activity. For instance, there may be a lead data manager when several data managers are involved. He or she coordinates within the sub-team, communicates with the trial manager and is accountable for the deliverable.

Communication, information sharing and follow up are important components of project management. All stakeholders need to be updated on the study progress to plan their work. It could be through periodic face to face meetings, teleconferences, or email communications. SharePoint, which can be accessed by all the members, could be used to update progress and register issues. Automated communication systems are also increasingly in use for notifications and reminders. The trial managers or other responsible personnel should ensure the readiness of team members to take up the next activity swiftly at a given time. When faced with issues, which may affect activities of other stakeholders, it should be effectively communicated.

Trial managers should have a broad understanding of the processes of various activities and sub-teams. At periodic intervals, critical paths of the entire trial and dependencies of individual activities should be reviewed. Risk identification and contingency planning are helpful, as most trials would face some challenges during operation. Preparedness and deliverable of each team member are important for smooth progress and meeting critical milestones. Lastly, motivating the team and keeping the morals high is vital.

Several computer programs are available to help project management in clinical trial operation. These are helpful to chart the entire trial, find dependencies, understand critical paths as well as visualize the impact of any change. The progress of the trial can be also monitored easily utilizing these tools. Typically, any change to the project plan from the baseline plan is tracked. Tables and graphs can be extracted to present various aspects of trial planning and progress using these tools. In general, these are very helpful in large trials; however, it may be of limited use in smaller trials.

16.Stakeholder management in clinical trial

In the setting of clinical trials, stakeholders could be a very wide group of people within or outside the organization. The functions directly involved in trial conduct are the usual stakeholders. Besides, there could be other stakeholders depending on the business model.

A clinical trial is a complex endeavor of several people often indirectly linked in a matrix environment. They are often from different education, training, functional domain, expertise, organization, nationality, language, and interest, especially in multi-center and multi-country trials. Stakeholder management and effective communication are crucial for successful trial management. It is normal to have team members with differing priorities, work culture and expectations. Careful planning and effective communication bring them on board for the common purpose.

A clinical trial includes several activities, which may be conducted in sequence or parallel and may be interdependent. For instance, timely drug supply by the manufacturing team is crucial for a trial to begin; however, it is dependent on the timely forecast from the trial team. Understanding stakeholders, their work practice, dependencies, constraints, and timelines are necessary. Most organizations employ a project manager when several personnel or organizations are involved.

In a highly specialized environment, different people are involved in multiple projects at a time. Typically, the focus is on projects, which are of high priority in a top-down approach (as per upper management directions). Hence, the challenge is to have everyone on the same page or bring a similar level of attention from all the stakeholders when a project is not of high priority.

As several activities should run in a coordinated fashion, organizations develop processes and standard timelines to complete each activity. Resource planning is also necessary in terms of manpower, goods, and services. Due to the sheer number of external and internal factors as well as the nature of the business, priorities may change over time. For instance, a delay in health authority approval may delay the downstream activities of a trial. In such a situation, if a trial result is critical, a project, which was started as a non-priority one, could get into a pressure situation. While working on a high priority project, where extra-ordinary efforts are needed, it may be worthwhile to take upper management into confidence. It helps in better stakeholder management.

While planning a trial or any specific activity, all concerned stakeholders (internal or external) should be consulted and any outstanding issues should be resolved through agreement. The difference in opinion may arise with the study design, timelines, service provider selection, or data interpretation and so on. However, a constructive discussion with the logical and pragmatic approach is key to consensus building; it also keeps the motivation and commitment of the team. Imposing a plan may be counterproductive and should be avoided except in exceptional circumstances. Timely information to the stakeholders on the trial progress enables effective planning of respective activities. Proactive communication and alignment go a long way in stakeholder management.

17. Trial management beyond the written code

The clinical trials are big endeavors for sponsors, CROs and clinical sites in a true sense. The project managers play a critical role like a chief executive in a company and navigate through a variety of issues and complex active interplay of people, interests, requirements, regulations, business models and priorities. Clinical trial managers need the attitude and skill to demonstrate situational leadership for success. This topic will focus on the realities and general unwritten code of the clinical trial industry relevant to trial managers.

Clinical research is highly regulated to protect the health of subjects and data integrity. There is a heavy burden of regulations, guidance, processes, protocol, workflows, practices, etc. Most organizations have developed processes, business models, and practices to manage situations in an efficient, transparent, and predictable manner. However, despite all these, it is common to get into uncharted waters.

Clinical trials are multifunctional efforts with representation from various functions in a company. Each function is a stakeholder with some area of expertise or control over certain processes. While a project manager needs to deal with several stakeholders, every stakeholder is not a decision maker or equally influential. For instance, a drug supply manager need not decide if there should be a change in the control arm of the study. Nevertheless, the viewpoint of a drug supply manager is important to understand the implications of such changes. If there likely to be any issues in obtaining the comparator products, the decision making will consider those.

Arguably, the most important stakeholder for trial project managers is the function that owns the strategy, designs the trial, and obtains funding and ultimately the end user of the trial results. Each trial advances the clinical development plan of the investigational product; hence, it is critical to be able to forge a good working relationship with the functional representative of clinical development to understand the context of the trial and key scientific expectations from the trial.

Although most organizations have a business model, people may not stay in organizations too long to fully understand or follow it. The wider trial team often includes people from divergent functions, organizations with a different background, culture, training, experience, and expectations. Unique work cultures are naturally shaped by such individuals with considerable influence of priorities of the organization and attitudes of senior management.

There is another set of dynamics with personnel of the vendor organization. There may be several vendors each with a project manager or a similar point of contact. Understanding the work culture of vendor organizations is helpful.

Each trial comes with a unique scenario and a set of people to work with. Each member of the trial team has different interests, perspectives, and stakes in a trial. A team member who may show a lot of interest and attention may not have the right experience while a very experienced team member may be too busy for an unimportant trial. The relationship among the senior managers of each function may have considerable influence in the team dynamics.

Often there is not a perfect business model or a set of processes for smooth trial conduct. It is natural to get less than perfect support from some of the functions or the vendors. Most team members do not fully understand the big picture, the sequence of events in trial operation or the dependencies on key deliverables. The key expectations from a trial manager are to hold the broader team together and deliver the trial with the available resources. It is common that a trial manager is often a junior member in the organizational hierarchy; nevertheless, one must be able to demonstrate leadership even when working with some senior members of the organization.

To command respect, a trial manager needs to fully understand the end to end processes and have a clear knowledge of ongoing activities, trial metrics or key issues. While striving to create a positive environment for the team members to contribute, ability to hold people accountable in a friendly manner is necessary. Ability to influence stakeholders is a key strength desirable for trial managers. Not all interactions are expected to be pleasant but outright conflicts should be avoided through available mechanisms. A trial manager should be on top of things and demonstrate leadership of the project through understanding, actions, and communications.

Trial teams are increasingly global and team members operate from different geographic locations remotely in different time zones. Hence, there are fewer opportunities for face to face interactions and informal relationship building. This is a unique challenge to a trial manager to understand diverse cultures, people, issues, key stakeholders and figure out the best ways to manage different circumstances. Communication skills are crucial in this context to be able to influence the right people at the right time. Emails, while the most common mode of communication, it is not the best way to influence people. Informal face to face or phone conversations are typically more effective.

Awareness of key areas of focus at various stages of the trial is crucial. Major milestones of the trial need proactive planning to avoid firefighting scenarios. The key dependencies, the involvement of individual team members and any risk should be carefully thought about. The trial manager should plan, discuss, communicate, and update the team continuously to be effective in achieving milestones. Many people need to be reminded or clarified about their responsibilities and the role of the trial manager becomes crucial in that respect.

While working with both internal and external stakeholders, the expectations or deliverables should be made clear and it should be reminded periodically. Irrespective of individual motivations, most people like to see their contributions in a positive way and nobody likes to be perceived to be standing in the way of a key deliverable of an organization. Mapping the details in granular details with constant monitoring and communication are some of the ways to influence stakeholders to perform.

Setting the priorities in the context of the big picture and organizational expectations is often crucial. Too often, timelines and budget are the points of focus while the quality of the trial is taken for granted. Budget and timelines are often set internally and can be modified while inferior quality work may cause irreparable damage. Although trial managers are responsible to operate within approved budget or timelines, those are determined internally and can be modified. Trial managers should not make any compromises on quality to manage a trial within the budget or timeline.

Issues are common in trial operations. Some of those can be foreseen and avoidable. Many of the issues could be just minor and have no significant impact on the key deliverables and could be ignored. Ability to expect and proactively manage issues comes with experience but is also a key skill set. Consultation with experienced colleagues is helpful.

It is not possible to resolve every issue or have a mitigation plan for every risk. Stakeholder management in the face of significant challenges is crucial to avoid unnecessary distraction. It is not uncommon when some issues become intractable leading to considerable attention from superiors or senior management. Often, it is possible to get an early sign of the issues to prevent crises. For issues, which may have serious implications, it may be the right time to communicate that at an early stage. Addressing perceptions informally is helpful.

Escalations are not the best way to resolve issues but may be needed in some situations. Most organizations have informal ways for escalations to seek attention. Typically, the scientific owners of the trials initiate escalations when milestones are missed, or quality has been compromised. Trial managers when in need of more budget or time should work with scientific owners of the trials for effective lobbying with senior management prior to formal requests.

Working with vendors or external partners can be tricky and the motivations of vendor organizations could be complex. A trial manager may have little influence on the vendor in the context of one trial. Vendor organizations typically have little stakes in the ultimate outcome of one trial from a sponsor. The process and motivations to outsource work to a vendor could be multi-factorial and not influenced by one trial. Clarity on the scope of work, setting the expectations right at the outset, clear detailed guidance and constant monitoring are helpful. The aim should be to bring a sense of ownership and accountability. Blame games are unhelpful in the long term and escalations can serve at the best as short-term fixes.

Periodic trial team meetings could be a very effective forum for a trial manager. Successful engagement with stakeholders in this meeting is immensely crucial. Team members should be encouraged to actively take part and bring issues and updates freely. The goals, deliverables, and issues should be prioritized in the context of the big picture and everyone should see them part of the team. The format should be adapted periodically as necessary.

18. Resource planning and analytics

Resource and operation planning is important for clinical development programs as projects take several years and comprises of many trials. Information on standard metrics is crucial to efficient planning and projections. The metrics could be on timelines (e.g. regulatory approval time or recruitment time), budget (e.g. investigator fees, procedure costs) or operational elements (e.g. standard of care, screen failure rates, dropout rates, risk factors, etc). Traditionally, project managers have relied on historical data in the company, prior experience, or individual networks for such insights. Gradually, newer platforms that utilize data science technologies have evolved to offer data-driven insights.

A large amount of operational data captured in clinical trials by various sponsors over time from tens of thousands of trials has been aggregated in a confidential and anonymous manner to provide operational insights. Data can be aggregated as necessary by the phase of clinical development, therapeutic area, indication, country, etc. for custom requirements. Currently, several service providers offer such solutions to obtain operational insights for clinical trial planning.

Such insights or analytics cover wide range of topics. For instance, modules that cover investigator site related costs (based on fair market value concepts) are commonly in use especially in large-scale multi-country trials. While investigators may not always fully agree on budget proposals using such tools, nonetheless, it provides a good starting point to ensure fair and consistent site budget projections using industry benchmark data.

Insights and business intelligence in some other areas are extremely helpful in operational planning of trials such as information on clinical sites, recruitment timelines, screen failure rates, dropout rates, protocol deviations, safety reporting, country-specific standard of care, grant negotiation timelines, procedures covered by third-party insurers, monitoring requirements, etc.

Key performance indicator (KPI) in the context of trial operations is an important concept. These are measurable elements of operational performance, and it could be built around timelines, cost or quality. Certain standard metrics helps to compare performance with industry peers as well as that of contract research organizations (CROs) and sites. Different countries and clinical sites can be compared to for pragmatic site selection and enrolment planning. Hundreds of KPIs can be drawn out; however, it is important to identify the frequently used ones across the industry. KPIs on timeline and budget are often stressed upon in real life, while KPIs on quality are crucial to the overall success of the trial operation.

19.Oversight in outsourced trial

Outsourcing of trial activities to contract research organizations (CRO) is a new normal for pharma/biotech sponsors. The key driver of outsourcing is the minimization of R&D expenditures while navigating through peak and trough workloads. Operational elements are typically outsourced while organizations focus on core strategic areas. As the ultimate responsibility remains with the sponsor, oversight of outsourced activities is crucial to ensure deliverables meet expectations. Equally important is also to be able to demonstrate it in the event of an audit or inspection.

Delegated trial activities are categorized into functional areas such as trial planning, medical monitoring, regulatory, pharmacovigilance, data management, statistics, project management, drug supply, central laboratory, and monitoring. For objectivity, the outsourced trial activities, and the responsible person(s) within sponsor organizations to perform oversight are identified along with method, frequency, and documentation modality in a document such as a vendor oversight plan. It is a good practice to make such documents comprehensive without ambiguity. Clear identification of activities that remain with the sponsor personnel is essential.

The standard study documents serve as the reference documents for operational conduct of the trial by contracted organizations and those are identified in the oversight plan. Typically, these are the protocol, procedure manual, pharmacy manual, monitoring plan, medical monitoring plan, recruitment plan, data management plan, eCRF completion guidelines, data review plan, risk management plan, pharmacovigilance plans, serology or sample management plan, drug supply plan, site management plans, regulatory submission plans, trial document management plan, protocol deviation plans, etc. These documents also serve as the references for oversight.

Methods of oversight are detailed in the oversight plans or other similar documents. It could be by review of trial milestones, periodic trial updates, data listings, issue registers, protocol deviation listings, monitoring reports, trial metrics, different trial trackers, etc. Oversight activities are documented in specifically generated periodic reports or meeting minutes, email confirmations, issue registers, trial documents or trackers, etc. Typically, these documentations are filed in the trial master file (TMF).

The oversight method should ensure that the outsourced activities are performed and delivered under the triple constraints of the famous project management triangle i.e. budget, timelines, and scope (features and quality) forming the sides. As timelines and budget are more objective and are easily discernible, the scope is often compromised. It is not unusual to have situations with a compulsion to meet timeline or to manage within a given budget even though it might adversely affect quality. Functional representatives involved in oversight must carefully weigh the options in such tricky situations.

Sincerity, diligence, and accountability of the contracted organization make the oversight easier to manage while it is cumbersome otherwise. A considerable amount of work may spill over to the functional representatives trying to ensure quality when not performed by the CRO partners. It is a sensitive topic, and it should be carefully managed through the available alliance management processes.

20. Risk-based approach to clinical trial oversight and trial quality management

The ICH GCP guidelines published in 2016 (E6 R2, Step 4 version) acknowledges the impact the development and implementation of original ICG GCP (E6 R1) guideline had on the scale, cost and complexity of industry-sponsored clinical trials. Evolutions in technology and risk management processes offer efficiency with a greater focus on the relevant activities. The new guideline encourages implementation of a risk-based approach to all stages of a clinical trial process such as trial design, conduct, oversight, recording and reporting with a focus on human subject protection and reliability of trial results. A risk-based approach to quality management of clinical trials is a relatively new concept in clinical trial operations.

Quality management includes efficient, simple, operationally feasible trial protocol as well as clear, concise, and consistent operational documents. Tools and procedures for data capture and other information gathering are equally important. In a risk-based paradigm, the methods to ensure quality are proportionate to the risks. Here are the key components of such as approach:

- Critical process and data for human subject protection and data reliability are identified during protocol development

- Risk identification are considered at both system (i.e. SOP, personnel, computerized system, etc) and trial level

- Risk is evaluated based on likelihood of error occurrence, possibility of detection and impact on subject protection and reliability of trial results

- Risk control approaches are devised proportionate to the significance of the risk. It is necessary to keep specific risks below a predefined quality tolerance limits while certain risks could be accepted. Risk reduction activities are applied at various levels such as trial design, investigator and vendor selection, agreements defining roles and responsibilities, specific monitoring and training activities

- Risk communication involves documentation and effective communication of quality management activities to relevant parties to facilitate risk review and continual improvement.

- Risk review at periodic interval is a key component to assess if the quality management activities to control risks remain effective and relevant

- Risk reporting is an essential component of clinical study report to describe the quality management approach implemented along with deviations from the predefined threshold and remedial actions taken.

This newer approach envisages bringing more efficiency in a process driven manner with greater transparency. Risks to subject protection or data integrity can arise from sources often overlooked such as protocol development, vendor or site selection practices, investigator's workload, oversight approaches, clinical data review methods, etc. Trial quality management needs to be performed continuously at all stages of a trial i.e. planning, execution, and reporting. Documentation and communication are important components of quality management.

Risk-based monitoring also follows a similar principle; however, the scope of monitoring in the context of overall trial quality management is limited although significant. As such, monitoring is a specific part of the overall quality management plan in clinical trials.

21.Confidentiality management

Research and development bring innovative medicines, devices or diagnostic techniques to market and eventually generate revenue for healthcare companies. All such products are conceived, developed, and refined through research work, which is resource intensive with significant expenditures and finally creates information, which is intellectual property. Organizations that rely on innovation need to protect the intellectual property from competitors for survival.

In any organization, certain employees have access to the confidential information, which is also shared with external partners (e.g. service providers, investigators, monitors) during clinical trial conduct. Employees of the innovator company or service providers may potentially share this sensitive information with competitors or move to competitor organizations, thereby disseminate it. Hence, a legal framework is essential to protect sensitive information and confidentiality management is a cornerstone of such business.

Confidentiality agreement must be in place prior to any document sharing (e.g. protocol or investigator's brochure) with investigators, contract research organizations (CRO) and other service providers. Some organizations track each instance of document sharing with partners. Sponsors may provide computer systems for use by employees of service providers to minimize the potential distribution of information that can't be tracked.

Employment policies of research organizations may have strict confidentiality clauses (e.g. no work with competitor companies or similar projects in competitor companies for 2 years). Computer systems are typically configured with security systems to track any document transfer. Several restrictions may be enforced at the workplace such as access-controlled rooms, password protected computer systems, restricted use of the internet, the policy of no use external drives and restricted use of document databases to prevent unauthorized access or dissemination. Secured networks (e.g. VPN) are typically used to prevent hacking of network systems. However, creating awareness among the employees is key to effective confidentiality management.

Certain basic work culture such as locking the computer systems while not in use, proper handling of printed materials, prompt destruction of unnecessary printed materials and appropriate email practices helps in confidentiality management. Minimizing use of computers at public places (e.g. airports) or use with privacy screens and no discussion about work while outside office premises are few examples of expected behavior. Typically, employees are sensitized and periodically trained about confidentiality management and basic techniques to enforce it. Each employee must be aware of and follow the corporate policy of the organization on it.

While there is an inherent risk of proprietary information dissemination to competitors or other parties, too strict an approach in information sharing with the employees and stakeholders may hamper day to day functioning. It may create an unnecessary feeling of trust deficit and may vitiate the environment of team work. Similarly, while working with service providers or other partners, a framework must be developed for efficient information sharing while protecting company's intellectual property.

Confidentiality of certain information is also important in the context of maintaining blind of studies. There may be provisions for blinded and unblinded teams and the key principle to maintain blinding is an effective separation of information sharing. Typically, processes are established in terms of responsibility division, access control of information (i.e. both through physical barriers and electronic access control), communication between the teams and documentation of any breach.

22.Legal consideration in clinical trial

Certain documents in clinical research have direct legal implications. Undertakings, disclosures, agreements, declarations, and delegations are to name a few. The basic purpose of such documents is to certify compliance to rules and regulations, accountability to responsibilities or commitment to trial activities. These documents have legal status and should be prepared, approved, signed, and maintained appropriately and the responsible personnel should be aware of the implications. When necessary, the opinion of legal counsel of the organization should be taken.

Examples:

- Agreements between the sponsors and CROs or other service providers
- Investigator undertakings before the trial commences where he/she pledges to conduct the trial as per the regulations, GCP and protect the safety of the subjects
- Delegation of trial activities to other trial personnel while retaining the overall responsibility
- Financial disclosures by the investigator to declare his/her commercial interests in the sponsor that may create a conflict of interest
- Sponsor declaration about the drug product for custom purposes
- Declaration by investigator about the non-infectious nature of biological samples

Such documents must be understood and correctly completed, signed only by the responsible personnel and signatures should accompany dates. Some of these documents may be prepared in duplicates. Standard templates may be available from health authorities or other government authorities (e.g. financial disclosure or form 1572 of US FDA). Organizations typically have templates for many of these documents as per standard industry practices that take into consideration applicable regulations and legal framework.

Besides, legal clauses are present in other documents such as privacy or compensation clauses in consent forms, external disclosure clause in protocol or advertisement materials. Typically, organizations have standard texts in templates for different countries or regions confirming to country-specific requirements.

Often, there are circumstances to provide customary gifts to investigators as per cultural practices, reimburse site expenditure to support subject retention activities or purchase instruments to facilitate trial related work. There may be legal provisions with permissible limits on such expenditures or reporting requirements. Typically, organizations have internal policies to manage such scenarios. It is prudent to take legal opinion to comply with regulations.

23.Clinical trial team (CTT)

Drug development and specifically clinical trials require highly complex teamwork, as people from diverse backgrounds are involved in this intricate process. In academic settings, clinical research may be carried out by a small group of individuals who manage every step from planning to subject enrolment, sample collection to laboratory work, data collection to statistical analysis and report writing.

In the industry setting, such a model has given way to specialized units at various levels, focused on specific tasks, driven by processes, and often not aware of the broader perspective. The trial team size has grown considerably over the years, as the role of the sponsor is increasingly limited to planning, coordination and data interpretation, while most of the execution is undertaken by specialized service providers.

Every drug development program has experts at the program level from various backgrounds such as medicine, pharmacokinetics (PK), pharmacogenomics, toxicology, pharmacovigilance, regulatory, preclinical, biomarker, bio-pharmaceutics, statistics, software programming, drug supply management, finance, and project management. Each clinical trial is conceived at the program level during drug development or lifecycle management. There could be several trials planned at any given time for a compound. A program level leadership team drives the entire development of the compound, while each trial is run by a trial team. There is no standard naming convention for the roles or designations of a trial team and may widely vary among organizations.

A trial manager or operation leader is responsible for the overall operational delivery of a trial. The trial manager of a sponsor serves as the single point of contact and drives trial planning, conduct, and report preparation while coordinating with various stakeholders. Depending on the scale of a trial, the trial manager may be supported by additional associates.

A medical expert provides medical inputs to trial planning and is responsible for safety, efficacy and pharmacodynamics aspects of the compound under evaluation. Medical experts play key roles in trials where the primary objective is safety or efficacy (e.g. tolerability, therapeutic exploration, therapeutic confirmation, etc).

A pharmacokineticist is responsible for pharmacokinetics (PK) aspects of the compound under evaluation and plays a leading role in PK endpoint trials such as bioequivalence, bioavailability, and drug-drug interaction trials. Typically, substantial proportions of early drug development trials have PK endpoints. A biostatistician is responsible for basic trial design, sample size determination, and data analysis.

The above team members often form the core trial team and are involved in the overall development of a compound. They are involved from the time of trial conceptualization to the study report. Any significant decision on the trial is taken by the core team in consultation with the upper management. One of these members may be the trial team representative who updates the upper management on the progress.

A data manager is responsible for collecting the trial data generated at the clinical sites or laboratories. Data management involves case record form (CRF) designing, database programming and data clean up; it ensures availability of clean trial data in the database before database lock (DBL). A statistical programmer develops software programs for data analysis and statistical output generation.

A regulatory manager advises on the regulatory environment, requirements in terms of documentation and data for conducting a trial as well as handles communications and dealings with health authorities. He or she also represents the sponsor organization at the health authorities.

A pharmacovigilance expert has a key role in inputs on safety data generation, management, regulatory reporting, and oversight on compound safety.

Depending on the evaluations planned in a trial, experts in various domains are involved such as bio-analysis, pharmacogenetics, biomarker, electrophysiology, imaging, and so on.

A drug supply representative is responsible for planning and supply of investigational drugs including placebo and comparative drugs. He or she may also handle randomization and blinding aspects of a trial along with the statistician. Other experts help in setting up the interactive response technology (IRT) for randomization and blinding. A medical writer helps the trial team in writing the scientific trial documents such as protocol, investigator's brochure, scientific regulatory documents, consent forms, study reports, etc.

Quality is an integral part of every trial related activity to maintain credibility and integrity. Quality assurance and control representatives have specific roles and are involved as required.

Many of the trial related activities are increasingly outsourced to service providers. Hence, representatives from outsourcing, legal, finance, and accounting are involved in the identification of service providers, competitive bidding, negotiation, contract execution, and invoice payment.

Organizations usually have internal scientific bodies to review trial design, methodology, rationale, appropriateness, and scientific content during the trial planning and conduct. External experts or regulatory bodies may be consulted in cases of sensitive and important trials to ensure external acceptability. Safety data monitoring committees may be set up to monitor trials on an ongoing basis.

Investigator and the clinical site staff are responsible for the actual conduct of a trial in human subjects as well as coordination with the ethics committee. Typical activities are obtaining ethics committee approval of the trial, subject recruitment, drug administration and clinical assessment. The site staff may include study coordinator, pharmacists, nurses, subject recruitment specialists and other specialized team members. Clinical sites work with local laboratories for medical investigations in the trial. Laboratories also have various staff such as project manager, lab director, analyst, data manager and quality control/assurance representatives.

Sponsors typically appoint field monitors to observe and review study conduct at clinical sites to ensure that the study is conducted as per the protocol and regulations. Managing trial supplies (medicinal products, ancillary supplies, laboratory kits, etc) requires specific expertise in planning, logistics and international regulations on cross border shipments and various services are required in this process (e.g. drug and sample shipment, storage). Several specialized courier agencies have evolved to cater to these needs.

There are other roles to support documentation, regulatory dossier preparation, trial portal management, translations, trial disclosures, and communications and so on depending on the complexity of the trial.

A broad outline of different roles in a clinical trial is described here. However, depending on the business model, the roles and responsibilities could be more specific or broader.

24. Multi-country and multi-center clinical trial

Clinical trials in patients or healthy subjects are generally conducted in multiple centers to meet recruitment goals. Usually, trials are planned in countries where market access is intended; however, it may not be the case all the time. A typical trial in a phase III program may require more than two thousand subjects depending on the nature of the disease condition and endpoints. Early development trials require less number of subjects but the intensity of evaluations and follow up may be higher. Currently, multi-country trials are the norm, rather than an exception. Nevertheless, conducting these trials pose unique challenges due to the interplay of different regulatory environments, cultures, and healthcare practices.

Typically, recruitment rate per month and cost per patient at an average site in different countries in specific disease indications are available from earlier trials. This is often the guiding principle to decide the number of sites in any country based on the projected available recruitment time. Several factors are taken into consideration for deciding the countries or sites for a trial conduct. Regulatory requirement/environment, commercial interest, patient availability, ease of recruitment, cost, standard of care, experience of investigators/sites, facility at the sites, regulatory compliance, ethnicity, and compliance to international disease management guidelines are some of the important considerations.

The regulatory environment is a key driver of clinical trials in a country or region. Faster review timeline, streamlined process, and minimal documentation requirement encourage preference of certain countries over others. There may be regulatory requirement to have a certain percentage or number of trial subjects from a particular country for product approval. Trials with longer recruitment or follow up duration are not significantly affected by a long approval time. Database of country-specific requirements and approval timelines are generally maintained by organizations for quick evaluations. If there are unique requirements, which are difficult to meet, the particular country selection could be affected.

Higher prevalence of a disease under study is particularly attractive. In addition to the availability of patient population, other key determinants are ease of conducting trials, experience of investigators, standard of practice (diagnostic tools used, the standard of treatment, follow up practices, etc.), co-morbidities in the patients, cost and quality in a given country. International guidelines may not be followed leading to difficulty in protocol implementation. Lifestyles, food habits, language and cultural practices are also taken into consideration. Information about the experience on similar trials provides important operational insight about different countries and sites.

Apart from regulatory and subject related factors, the adherence to study protocol is an important consideration. Commercial reasons such as the intended countries of market access could play a key role in country selection in late phase trials. Certain key opinion leaders may have to be considered as investigators in a region and it could drive country selection.

While developing a protocol, feedback from different sites or countries improves feasibility. However, too many suggestions or conflicting suggestions are hard to implement. A strategy to consider inputs from coordinating investigators of different countries or regions may be more practical. In many instances, the protocol is developed with the help of few investigators, and then, investigators from other countries or sites are included based on feasibility of implementation.

A draft synopsis is often used to seek suggestions before drafting the protocol. Different health authorities and ethics committees may suggest conflicting modifications to the protocol. Site and country-specific amendments may be considered when it is feasible and does not change the overall trial conduct or study population. It is an important consideration for the country and site selection.

Investigational product related requirements could be significantly different in terms of availability of comparator drugs, country-specific data requirements, storage and dispensing conditions or labelling and must be evaluated during trial planning. Biological sample or drug shipment requirements may differ in different countries. Translation of study documents to local language is needed in certain countries for review by regulatory authorities, ethics committees and site staff. Timelines and cost of translation must be taken into consideration.

The service providers in the trial should be evaluated for their ability to cater to all the planned countries or sites. Some service providers may have arrangements with other sub-contractors for operations at certain locations. Certain service providers may have teams in different countries for cost or resource optimization. Data management, safety data processing, medical writing, and laboratory evaluations in many global trials are often managed remotely far away from the sites of trial conduct. Logistics and human aspects of centrally or remotely managed trial activities should be considered.

The trial team set up should support global connect with the development program while maintaining local operational efficiency and knowledge. Differences in language, work culture, working hours, holiday schedule, etc. should be managed with sensitivity. Expectations, requirements, and problems at different sites or countries may be unique. Some sites may need support for equipment while others may have issues with trained personnel. In some countries, the regulatory approval could be faster, while recruitment is slower.

Pharmacovigilance operations in multiple countries with unique reporting requirements could be challenging. Any safety issues from one site or country have to be appropriately communicated to the other participating sites as per regulations. Document archival requirements may vary at different sites or countries. Subject confidentiality or privacy regulations may be different, so also could be publications or postings of trials and results in public forums.

Project management tools are imperative to keep track of progress at multiple countries and sites. Crucial activities such as recruitment, drug supply, monitoring, biological sample management, data entry, etc. need to be continuously tracked. Recruitment and retention issues could be diverse from under recruitment at some sites to over recruitment at others. A recruitment and retention plan helps to set the expectations including the desired proportion of enrolment in participating countries and plan for reallocation in the event not meeting goals. Often, investigators are unhappy when their recruitment targets are reduced even if they have difficulty in meeting it; cultural sensitivities should be taken into consideration.

Periodic engagement with service providers and investigators could be challenging and periodic updates, newsletters, teleconferences or face to face meetings are necessary to maintain team spirit. A healthy competitive environment could be created among the sites to recruit subjects and deliver quality data. There should be clarity and understanding on the issues that could be discussed in groups or on a one to one basis.

Optimization of trial sites and resources are typically necessary during the trial. Non-performing sites could be dropped while new countries or sites are added.

25. Clinical trial protocol

The protocol is defined in ICH GCP as "A document that describes the objective(s), design, methodology, statistical considerations, and organization of a trial. The protocol usually also gives the background and rationale for the trial, but these could be provided in other protocol referenced documents". The protocol is the most important document in the context of a clinical trial.

A protocol has both technical and administrative information, which the sponsor determines to be necessary for a trial from recruitment of subjects to report generation. Health authorities, ethics committees, and other concerned authorities review and approve the protocol before its implementation. The investigators must follow the protocol to conduct the trial. The monitors verify that the trial conduct is according to the protocol. Finally, data analysis and report preparation are also performed as per the protocol. Typically, there is a synopsis with a concise description of the most essential and high-level elements of the protocol.

Protocol development is a multifunctional teamwork and involves an iterative process of review, consultation, and refinement. A protocol development team under the leadership of a clinical development representative is generally the norm in an industry setting. Individual team members with specific expertise are responsible for specific sections of the protocol. Often, a medical writer is responsible for managing the content and formatting, and drafts the first version from a concept sheet taking inputs from the trial team. It is not unusual to have team members commenting on sections, which are not their domain of expertise. It is essential that individual members are aware of their specific responsibilities for efficient teamwork.

Initiation of many trial operations activities is linked to the availability of a draft protocol or synopsis such as feasibility evaluation, budget estimation, site identification, data management plan, etc. and feedback from health authorities or external experts where appropriate. Subsequently, a final protocol is the basis to finalize many study documents or trial plans such as the case report form (CRF), informed consent form (ICF), monitoring plan, drug supply plan and statistical analysis plan. Many such activities have varying lead times from a final protocol and need to be considered.

Similarly, any change to the study protocol needs the revision of several other documents or plans and could potentially affect the timelines, budget or quality. Typically, most study documents are initiated based on a synopsis or draft protocol and those are formally finalized after the protocol is final. It is important to balance the dependent activities and take into consideration all factors potentially affecting the protocol.

Discrepancies in different sections of the protocol are one of the common reasons for protocol amendment or clarification notes. It is a good practice not to repeat any information in different sections, rather writing it in the most appropriate section and referring to it in other relevant sections. For instance, a sample collection schedule could be specified only in the assessment schedule, which is referred to throughout the protocol. Using an access controlled document management system with write access to few authors and quality checks at the end are few other steps to minimize errors.

Lack of clarity or ambiguity in the protocol leads to differing interpretation and is a commonly observed problem. Procedures, assessments, and entry or withdrawal criteria descriptions in the protocol should be as simple as possible. Proactive discussion with the investigators, pharmacists, laboratory personnel at the site and other stakeholders for appropriate interpretation at the draft stage is helpful. Interpretation by a colleague not involved in the study could be useful.

Often investigators and site staff come up with feasibility issues in the protocol at later stages (i.e. at the time of site initiation) unaware of the fact that there is little flexibility once the protocol is final and approvals are in place. Pragmatic trial planning should consider proactive discussions with investigators (as possible) at early stages to take practical insights. Especially, study eligibility criteria, key evaluations, standard of care measures and extent of follow up evaluations should be considered from a ground reality perspective. It may be safe to presume that the site staffs have not understood the protocol unless it has been specifically discussed with them.

In general, a protocol should be as flexible as possible without compromising scientific principles. Strict protocols that provide little flexibility lead to protocol deviations or necessitate future amendments. For instance, strict laboratory ranges for eligibility criteria or strict assessment windows for evaluations when not necessary would be difficult to follow in a trial. A follow-up visit after 2 months interval without any window period may be difficult to achieve in reality, while a window period of +/- 3 days would be more practical for such a visit. Restrictions for subjects that are not necessary should be avoided in the protocol.

Too many inputs or reviews to protocol make it a never-ending process. There should be a clear plan or process for the protocol review. It is ideal to discuss conflicting issues in meetings rather than in email communications. Deadlines should be set and respected. Inputs from all investigators in a multicenter trial may be counterproductive. However, key investigators should be involved at an earlier stage. Once the protocol is final, many downstream activities are triggered. Changes to the protocol can be made only through an official amendment, as version control is the norm.

70

Certain amendments to subject safety, evaluations, duration of follow up or entry criteria may need health authority or ethics committee approval before implementation. However, in emergencies, changes can be implemented in the interest of subject safety while approvals are pending. Depending on the organizations, health authorities or ethics committees, an amendment could be a time consuming and cumbersome process. Protocol amendment may also trigger amendments to ICF, CRF, monitoring plan, contracts, budgets, etc.

In an alternate approach, the protocol could be developed as a concise document through limiting the operational content. This improves readability of the document with concise but enough information for regulatory review while some of the operational details are elaborated in separate protocol referenced documents such as procedure manual, laboratory manual, pharmacy manual, recruitment plans, etc. In general, competent authorities or ethics committees do not review or approve these documents. Such an approach provides more flexibility and is consistent with ICH GCP guidance, which allows some of the protocol content to be in other documents. Many of the procedural details are typically available closer to trial initiation and are common reasons for protocol amendment.

26. Copy, paste, template and translation error

Clinical trials are documentation intensive and numerous documents are generated in the course of a trial conduct. Protocols, informed consent form, monitoring plan, statistical analysis plan, subject file, clinical study report, drug forecast form, vendor worksheet, initiation visit slides are to name a few.

Typically, people working on a project refer to previous such documents and copy-paste sections from one document to another or edit a previous such document. In multi-country and multi-center trials, country or site-specific documents are typically customized from global documents. While it helps to minimize duplicate efforts, error in previous documents or text not applicable to the new trial, may creep in inadvertently. Scientific document translations could pose challenges, as sometimes the nuances in the meanings are lost.

Such errors are relatively common and could lead to very troubling situations. Conflicting information may be discovered at the time of health authority review or trial conduct. It may lead to queries from health authorities on study protocols, reports or other regulatory documents. Considerable time and effort may be required to make amendments, provide clarifications or prepare file notes. Trial misconduct may arise due to such conflicting information.

A general level of awareness is crucial to address such issues to a considerable extent; most people with some years in the industry have some unpleasant experience because of such errors. In addition, several approaches such as peer review, checklists, innovative templates, proactive quality control (QC) for a list of common errors could be used.

Depending on the type of document and the time of identification, an appropriate approach could be adopted to rectify an error. It could be a clarification letter, file note, amendment, or response to a query and so on. If any trial misconduct has happened due to such an error, its impact should be evaluated along with the implementation of corrective actions.

To help in document development and standardization of content, most organizations have templates of various documents with detailed instructions. Typically, the templates have mandatory texts, which are required to be left as such or to be only modified with approval and texts to be customized as necessary for individual trial. While a good template is a great starting point, a bad template may create an inflexible situation, especially mandatory texts. Template issues should be brought to the notice of appropriate personnel and addressed in periodic reviews.

27.Subject eligibility criteria

Subject eligibility criteria are the characteristics of the population who may participate in a clinical trial. Generally, it is in the form of inclusion and exclusion criteria. The inclusion criteria must be met, and the exclusion criteria must not be present to fulfil eligibility. A combination of demographic, clinical history, physical examination, laboratory evaluation and lifestyle measures constitute the eligibility criteria with an objective to enrol a group of subjects who would represent the population to whom the trial outcome may be applicable. In the exploratory phase of drug development, eligibility criteria are designed to minimize variability and homogenize the trial population. In the later phase of drug development, eligibility criteria are relaxed to allow wider participation.

Fundamentally, while a set of restrictive criteria narrows the scope of trial outcome and ultimate applicability, a relaxed set of criteria broadens the scope; however, it may also create a situation where the scientific principle cannot be clearly demonstrated due to confounding factors. Investigators are required to adhere to the protocol selection criteria as it has substantial ethical, regulatory, scientific and safety implications. In each disease condition, the safety efficacy of a drug may not be similar across the population. It is essential to figure out a population where the efficacy is maximum with minimum safety concerns. In general, a drug gets approval for use in a population, which was evaluated in the confirmatory trials.

Eligibility criteria are framed in line with the study objective, disease condition, associated co-morbidities, concomitant medications and other practical considerations. Broadly, it consists of standard disease diagnostic criteria as well as acceptable health parameters based on history, clinical and laboratory evaluations. Lifestyle measures, comprehension of the trial, ability to comply with the protocol and ability to spare sufficient time for participation are important considerations. While dealing with healthy subjects, it is important to stipulate what can be considered healthy.

Restrictive criteria may pose a hindrance to trial conduct leading to poor recruitment, cost escalations, delay in trial completion, protocol amendments and loss of enthusiasm at the clinical sites. Timely review and consultation with the stakeholders can minimize this issue significantly.

Investigators' feedback should be taken into consideration before protocol finalization. Typically, the scientists working to decide the study population may not have precise information about the target population at different countries or clinical sites. Investigators could provide practical insights or any change in disease presentation in their locality. However, consultations with each investigator may be counterproductive in large trials. Difficulty in finding enough subjects could be managed by relaxing the entry criteria where possible or with effective preparedness in terms of a large number of good clinical sites and practical timelines.

Certain trials have a standard of care (SoC) as a comparator treatment arm and the investigational treatment arm as the new drug in addition to SoC. Some trials consider failure to SoC as an entry criterion. SoC may vary from country to country as well as among different hospitals in one country. Certain therapies are not universally available in all countries. Routinely used doses of standard drugs may vary in different countries.

Common co-morbid conditions in the target population should be considered. For instance, many subjects with diabetes may have hypertension and lipid abnormalities. Hence, it may be relatively difficult to find subjects with only diabetes without any co-morbidity. Similarly, patients with disease conditions may be under certain medications, which need to be considered. Looking for treatment-naive patients may be troublesome for recruitment. Innovative trial designs or flexibility in the allowed concomitant medications is conducive to trial feasibility where acceptable. Stratification of the subjects to different groups may be an option.

Social and cultural issues should be taken into consideration. For instance, it is difficult to enrol women in healthy volunteer trials in certain countries. Smoking is often cited as an exclusion criterion without any clear rationale; a particular intensity of use (e.g. > 10 cigarettes per day) is a more practical and logical criterion. With every additional criterion, the target population shrinks adding further difficulty. Each such criterion should be guided by strong scientific rationale.

Commonly, investigators or site personnel don't pay attention or appreciate the challenges until recruitment begins. Typically, investigators come up with questions about the eligibility criteria at the site initiation meeting or at the first opportunity when they pay close attention. However, it is hardly possible at that time to make any modifications due to the operational complexities involved. Innovative and pragmatic ways to discuss the target population with the investigators could be helpful.

Organizations have protocol templates or previously conducted similar trials, which become the basis of newer ones. Many texts in the template or previous trial protocols may be taken for granted as standard, which may be impractical in the new context. Each trial should be looked at freshly in the light of the current circumstances.

Many health parameters can vary when repeated over a period. Protocol requirement to meet such variable clinical or laboratory parameters within a tight range at multiple visits in the run-up to randomization may be challenging. The protocol should be flexible to allow entry into the trial based on clinical significance based on investigator's judgment of such parameters. Repetition to rule out laboratory error should be allowed.

A central laboratory for eligibility assessments is often used for reliability and uniformity. However, it may be logistically difficult at clinical sites. Sample shipment delays, holiday schedule, the convenience of subjects, the lag time of central laboratory reporting, and mode of communication may create challenging situations, especially at the time of baseline evaluation prior to study treatment initiation. Whenever possible, dependence on the central laboratories for eligibility evaluation should be minimized or sufficient lead time should be factored in.

Run-in period may be part of a protocol after screening and before the study treatment initiation. It is utilized for withdrawal or modification of background treatment, assessment of placebo response, familiarization to study procedures, stabilization of baseline health parameters, compliance assessment or eligibility confirmation. Unreasonable run-in period in a trial, especially that requires withdrawal or modification of previous medications could be unethical or unconvincing for subjects.

Diagnostic approaches of diseases may vary in different regions. For instance, X-ray of the chest is a common procedure to rule out tuberculosis in India whereas it is not the case in the western countries. Some health authorities or ethics committee may ask for additional safety evaluations to entry criteria. These factors should be considered during protocol development. Additional country-specific eligibility criteria may be added to the extent it does not affect the overall study population; however, the country-specific applicability should be clearly emphasized.

Method of eligibility criteria evaluation should be clarified in the protocol. It could be only based on clinical history, past records, physical or laboratory evaluations. For instance, it should be clarified whether a genetic test is needed to exclude a disease condition or only clinical history is sufficient. In case of laboratory evaluations, specific details on method, time and interpretation should be clarified without any ambiguity.

At the clinical site, a checklist is used for confirming eligibility at screening and baseline. Sites could be asked to prepare or provided with such a checklist. It lists down all eligibility criteria as in the protocol and an investigator verifies the subject records against the checklist to confirm eligibility. The checklist is also verified by the field monitor in the monitoring process.

28.Safety evaluation in clinical trial

Safety evaluations are part of clinical trials to assess eligibility and monitor adverse events due to investigational treatment. 'Safety evaluation' is a commonly used term and is understood as all such evaluations that are typically not used for typical endpoints in the trial such as pharmacokinetics, pharmacodynamics, biomarkers, pharmacogenetics, etc. However, it may not be entirely correct, and some investigations may serve as both. Safety evaluations broadly cover the following purposes:

- Subjects meeting eligibility criteria and otherwise healthy enter the study
- Co-morbidities of subjects are under control at the time of entry and during the trial conduct to minimize confounding factors
- Any adverse events due to trial participation are monitored and identified promptly

- Subjects meeting stopping rules are swiftly identified and withdrawn from the trial to safeguard their health
- If a trial has multiple stages (e.g. within group dose escalation), subjects are deemed eligible before entering the next stage
- Subjects leave the trial in good health or at the least the health status is known at that time

Examples of safety evaluations are clinical history, vital sign, physical examination, ECG, hematology, biochemistry, urinalysis, tests for substance abuse, chest X-ray, and ultrasonography. Certain evaluations e.g. physical examination, hematology or biochemistry may have several test parameters depending on the requirement or standard practice.

Safety evaluations should be planned appropriately to the profile of the compound, experience, and biological plausibility. The evaluations may also depend on the disease condition or type of study (exploratory vs. confirmatory, clinical pharmacology vs. safety/efficacy evaluation, etc.). Inadequate evaluations may jeopardize the subject safety and underestimate adverse events. Intense assessment schedule or too many procedures are a stress on recruitment or retention, trial logistics, protocol compliance and overall trial budget.

Whenever possible, invasive biological fluid collections and evaluations should be minimized. If acceptable, there should be flexibility in prerequisites for safety samples. For instance, random blood glucose could be considered instead of fasting blood glucose. Many tests can be performed at any time of the day rather than in the morning hours or in fasting condition. However, if a restriction or preparation is necessary for proper assessment, it should be followed.

Visit schedule should be planned considering the turnaround time of the safety laboratory. Typically, sites use their own local laboratory for routine tests. When a central laboratory is used, the turnaround time may be longer. It may be worthwhile to keep a wider window for baseline evaluations rather than just a day prior to randomization. Certain assessments such as 24-hour Holter ECG or a pharmacogenetic test at a central laboratory may take several days for evaluation and reporting. Microbiology culture reports may take a couple of days or some tests as such may need a longer time in the normal course. The logistics of equipment requirements, shipment, evaluations, and reporting should be taken into consideration.

Choice of central or local laboratory for each safety parameter evaluation should be clarified in the protocol. Generally, central laboratories are preferred for the reliability of data, standardization of evaluations across trial sites or feasibility issues at the local laboratories. In case of emergency, when the use of a central laboratory may be impractical, local laboratory use may be allowed for operational efficiency. Many of these issues should be foreseen and thought out in advance to prevent confusion during trial conduct.

Case report form (CRF) should be designed according to the need to collect safety data into the database for analysis. All safety data is not required for analysis and hence, need not be collected. Certain evaluations are only necessary for safety monitoring at the clinical site by the investigators. Typically, there are provisions in the CRF to collect data from both planned and unplanned safety evaluations.

Information about the proportion of subjects with abnormal tests in the target study population could be obtained from the laboratories, investigators, and previous trials and are helpful to understand expected screen failure rates. Normal ranges of tests should be pragmatically decided to take into consideration local factors. Decisions could be left to investigators with a broad guidance or with provisions for consultation with sponsor's medical monitor. However, too many case-by-case decisions could be impractical in large trials.

During a new compound development, several clinical trials are conducted to evaluate safety and efficacy. Often considerable effort is wasted to finalize appropriate safety assessments and its frequency. Building a generic safety evaluation panel for a compound is a practical approach to minimize duplicate efforts. This could be then customized to individual trials as necessary.

The sequence of assessments at screening and baseline while evaluating eligibility should be carefully planned at the site considering practical aspects such as convenience and cost of tests. For instance, evaluations of history and physical examination may be performed before blood collections or other invasive procedures. It ensures subjects who are not eligible based on simpler assessments don't undergo invasive procedures.

Country or region-specific evaluations for certain disease diagnoses may exist. Health authorities or ethics committees may request additional safety evaluations, which may have to be considered locally. Site or country-specific protocol provisions could be made in such cases. Flexible protocol language such as 'Test A-may be conducted as per local guidance' may be used. However, significant changes to the over-all eligibility should not be allowed as it may introduce variability in the study population.

Safety evaluations may break the blind in a blinded study due to the predictable pharmacologic effect of investigational drugs. For instance, certain drugs may decrease lymphocyte counts, increase pulse rate, decrease blood pressure, decrease blood glucose level, or have an effect on other physiologic parameters, which are routinely part of safety assessments. Appropriate planning is essential to handle such safety data at the clinical site. One possible solution is to have an unblinded or independent investigator to perform such clinical evaluations or to be notified about such laboratory parameters. Alternatively, the laboratory may be instructed not to report such parameters to the investigator unless a specified threshold is breached. Data management activities need to be planned accordingly such as having an independent staff to enter such information in the CRF.

Clinical significance of abnormalities should be noted in the subject file and reported in case report form (CRF). Any abnormal parameter unless deemed clinically insignificant, would be considered protocol deviation (deviation to eligibility criteria) before randomization or adverse event (AE) after randomization. The investigator is particularly responsible to determine the clinical significance and report adverse events. Any abnormal value deemed clinically insignificant (where there are no predefined ranges in the protocol) must be explicitly documented in the source document. It should also be reported in the comment section of the CRF.

Many lab parameters may have different normal ranges at different regions depending on the population and laboratory. The normal values for such parameters are typically not specified in the protocol. In specific situations, cut off values may be described in the protocol for uniformity. If a test result is outside the normal range, laboratory errors may be ruled out by repeating the test. The procedure for repeating a test (when, where, how many times or what is acceptable out of the repeat test) should be specified in the protocol. For instance, the protocol may allow an abnormal test result reported from the central laboratory for serum potassium to be repeated locally in borderline cases and if it is normal, appropriate decisions may be made accordingly. Some tests when abnormal need to be repeated only after an interval of time.

Laboratory parameters may be altered in disease states and normal range of laboratories may not be applicable in such situations. Acceptable limits of laboratory parameters may vary in different physiological and pathological conditions. Such issues should be addressed in the protocol by providing acceptable ranges. Sponsor's medical expert should review the laboratory normal ranges prior to trial initiation and periodically in a long-term trial.

Generally, abnormal tests during the study if considered clinically significant qualify for AE reporting. In such cases, the subject might have to be followed up until the values return to normal or remain unchanged. Abnormal parameters considered clinically insignificant are not usually followed up. However, some ethics committees or local authorities might require follow up of such values as well if outside the normal range. The follow-up plan should be clarified in the protocol or other study documents.

AEs may occur due to non-compliance to study restrictions. For instance, a protocol dealing with a drug inducing hypotension might have a restriction on getting up from bed for some hours after drug administration. Inability to follow that may lead to accidental falls. Inability to take food at advised times might lead to hypoglycemia in trials evaluating drugs with glucose-lowering potential. Subjects should be advised properly on that. The trial could be planned in a way to prevent such events. For instance, domicile stay may be planned for adequate supervision.

Investigators may conduct additional investigations or evaluations, which were not planned in the protocol, in the interest of the safety of trial subjects. In general, it is allowed from a GCP standpoint on the ground of subject safety; investigators need not seek any authorization from the sponsor in such situations.

29. Pharmacokinetics (PK) evaluation

Clinical trials such as bioavailability, bioequivalence, drug-drug interaction, food effect, pharmacokinetics (PK) in a special population (renal and hepatic failure) evaluate PK parameters as the primary objective. In some other cases such as PK/PD, tolerability (first in man single and multiple ascending dose trials) and thorough QT trials, PK remains an important secondary endpoint. PK may be part of a trial trying to understand population PK, where sources and correlates of variability in drug concentrations in the target patient population are investigated. Sometimes, limited PK samples may be taken to assess treatment compliance.

Generally, PK studies are conducted in healthy subjects unless there are safety concerns or compelling reasons to evaluate PK in a special or target population. In most situations, there is high predictability of data from healthy subjects to target patient populations. Study sample size largely depends on the design (crossover vs. parallel design), the variability of the compound in terms of PK parameters and study objective (e.g. drug-drug interaction study with a variable compound).

PK studies in healthy subjects are conducted in clinical pharmacology units (CPU), which are well organized and specialized settings. The entire study may be conducted at one go or in cohorts depending on the capacity of the CPU and recruitment rate. Many contract research organizations (CRO) have capabilities to run a trial in 50-60 subjects, at the same time.

PK of compounds may be influenced by lifestyle measures and such studies typically have intensive blood collection schedule; thus, domiciled stay at the CPU helps to maintain uniformity and is convenient for subjects. To facilitate domiciled stay and minimize any impact on work schedule, the domiciled period could be planned during weekends. Sites also plan recreational activities as permissible to keep subjects engaged during the stay. Two to four days of domiciled stay are usual; requirements for prolonged domiciled stay may lead to recruitment challenges. However, trials involving 3-4 weeks of the domiciled period have been reported in the literature.

Restriction on food or water intake, lifestyle measures, concomitant medication or posture is generally observed for PK evaluations. The requirement is specified in the protocol and subjects are explicitly informed about it during the informed consent process. Compliance with restrictions is evaluated and ensured through clinical history, counselling, reminders, laboratory tests and direct observation. It is noted in subject files and sometimes reported in CRF. The PK evaluation may be performed after drug administration in fasting or fed condition.

In food-effect studies, stipulated meal as per regulatory requirement is the norm.

Proper and timely drug administration is critical to accurate PK evaluation. Drug administration is typically supervised, and a mouth check is performed to verify that the subject has swallowed the formulation. Certain formulations should not be chewed prior to swallowing (e.g. modified release formulations); it must be clearly mentioned in the protocol and the subjects should be instructed accordingly.

When multiple drugs are to be administered at the same time, the sequence and time window (within which all the pills must be taken) should be clarified. Time of the day for drug administration (e.g. 8-10 AM in the morning) is kept uniform and all subjects are dosed within the same allowed time interval; individual subjects are dosed at the same time of the day in different periods of a crossover study to the extent possible. Any issues encountered during drug administration need to be noted in the subject files and reported in the comment section in case report form (CRF).

The biological sample to be collected for drug level estimation, time points, volume, the collection procedure, labelling, processing instruction, storage and transport conditions should be specified in the protocol or in a separate manual. All these aspects must be discussed with the site at the time of site feasibility evaluation and discussed with the concerned site staff at the time of trial initiation. Sample labelling is critical for accurate sample identity. Instruction for labelling should be provided in the protocol or in a separate manual. Barcode labels are commonly in use increasingly and may help to maintain blind in a blinded trial. Generally, PK data after bioanalysis is transferred from bioanalytical laboratory to the analysis database electronically.

The sample collection time is calculated from the drug administration time. Drug levels may be very sensitive to time of sample collection, especially if a compound has short half-life for absorption, distribution or excretion. In PK data analysis, the actual time of sample collection is considered; thus, it should be recorded and reported in the CRF irrespective of the scheduled or planned time. If multiple assessments coincide at one-time point (e.g. PK collection, BP measurement, ECG, etc), the protocol should have clear instruction on the sequence of priority based on scientific and logistic reasons. In many countries, standard times change during winter and summer leading to changes in post-dose timeframes in the middle of a trial; it should be foreseen.

Logistic considerations may not allow sample collection at the exactly planned time points. Acceptable time windows should be clearly stipulated for operational flexibility. The sampling times closer to dosing may have narrower windows, whereas later sampling times may have wider windows. On the days of intensive blood sample collection, indwelling catheters are preferred over multiple venipunctures. In the event of catheter blockade, collection via direct venipunctures is generally acceptable.

In the later part of PK sample collection schedule (terminal phase), a few sparsely scheduled samples may be collected in ambulatory visits. Thus, the subjects need not remain domiciled just for a couple of sample collections (e.g. 48 and 72 hours after dosing). Subjects can go back home and visit the site for these sample collections. Such arrangements may be more acceptable to subjects as it minimally disrupts their personal schedule and is cost effective. The protocol could be flexible to allow a prolonged domiciled stay if it is logistically more acceptable, especially for certain patient populations.

Vacutainers are typically used for precise blood volume draw using indwelling catheters. A normal syringe could also be used. To prevent blood clotting inside the indwelling catheter, heparin solution is typically injected; however, it may interfere with the analytical method of some compounds. Similarly, analytical methods of compounds may have compatibility issues with the anticoagulants used in the vacutainers. Sometimes, sourcing the desired tube of appropriate volume or with a particular anticoagulant may be an issue at the clinical site. This should be discussed and sorted out in advance.

Certain compounds are light sensitive, thereby require yellow monochromatic lighting systems at dosing, sample collection, and processing areas. Such facility should be confirmed with the site at the time of feasibility evaluation.

The most common biological fluid for drug level estimation is plasma; however, it could be whole blood, serum, urine, semen, milk, fat, saliva, peritoneal fluid, cerebrospinal fluid, etc. depending on study objective. In case of urine collections, time intervals (8-10 AM) rather than time points are planned to have adequate urine volume for sample collection.

Total volume or frequency of sample collection in a trial may raise ethical, safety or practical concerns from the site, ethics committee or health authority. For instance, upto 450 mL of blood collection, which is equivalent to the amount of collection in a voluntary blood donation, may be deemed safe in healthy subjects, although a higher volume may be acceptable if collected over a prolonged interval. It is prudent to follow country-specific guidance for better acceptability. There may be safety concerns with a higher frequency of cerebrospinal fluid (CSF) or tissue biopsy sample collection. It could be also discouraging for the potential subjects. Such issues should be proactively discussed with the investigators.

Route of drug administration may be different depending on the study objective and could be oral, subcutaneous, intravenous, sublingual, rectal or transdermal. Comparison of bioavailability after different routes of administration may be the study objective. Vomiting is an important consideration while drug administration is oral. Time of vomiting after administration, type of formulation and time to peak concentration of the compound are important considerations. Clear instructions should be provided on how to handle subjects who vomit after dosing.

30.Pharmacodynamics or efficacy evaluation

Pharmacodynamics (PD) is described as any pharmacological effect of a treatment on the pathophysiological process of the body. It can be measured in clinical or laboratory assessments. Several terminologies may be used to denote PD evaluations such as clinical, biochemical, pathological, electrophysiological, radiological, patient/physician reported outcome, pharmacogenomic or proteomic assessment that estimates drug effect on the body and is collectively described as PD evaluation.

It could be a measure of short-term or long-term effect and could involve a simple or complex procedure. Examples of PD evaluations are blood pressure, heart rate, lipid levels, TNF-alpha level, VAS score, EDSS score, muscle biopsy, MRI evaluation, QT interval, treatment success or failure, remission free survival, and death. While the desirable PD effects can be called efficacy, the undesirable effects are the adverse events (AE). Lack of efficacy or worsening of a body parameter can also be considered as a measure of efficacy. Many aspects discussed in the section on pharmacokinetics evaluation apply to this section.

These evaluations are of varying complexity from a procedural perspective. Fasting blood glucose, blood pressure or heart rate are examples of apparently simple assessments. Taking biopsy specimens, electroencephalograms, or positron emission tomography scans are some of the procedure intensive evaluations, which require special training and equipment. It could be cost and resource intensive as well.

Examples of studies where pharmacodynamics or efficacy endpoints are evaluated are therapeutic exploratory (such as proof of concept, dose ranging, PK/PD) and therapeutic confirmatory studies (efficacy endpoint). Such endpoints may be considered 'soft', where surrogate endpoints or biomarkers are used (e.g. BP in a hypertension trial or LDL in a lipid-lowering trial). This is often the case in therapeutic exploratory trials.

Efficacy endpoints are generally 'hard' endpoints such as an occurrence of stroke, death or myocardial infarction in a hypertension trial. Such endpoints are required in therapeutic confirmatory trials to provide unambiguous evidence of benefit. At this moment, only very few biomarkers are recognized as acceptable endpoints in therapeutic confirmatory trials for regulatory approval of new drugs.

Feasibility at the site is a key consideration, and it should be assessed during protocol development while planning such evaluations. In case of complex procedures, suitable site selection is crucial. Investigators or clinical sites with prior experience should be preferred. A clear understanding of the procedures and capability at the sites in terms of manpower, equipment, and infrastructure are important considerations. If it is difficult to identify appropriate sites, capacity building through funding for equipment, training, and investigator engagements may be considered. Often the site personnel underestimate the complexity of the procedures and end up with critical deviations.

Complex procedures should be stepwise detailed in a procedure manual with pictures or schematic diagrams to ensure clarity. Recorded video demonstrations may be useful when possible. Detailed information on the procedure is generally not required in the protocol. Keeping the details in a separate manual ensures faster protocol development and progress of downstream activities, which depend on a final study protocol. Finalization of many procedures goes through an iterative process of review and refinement involving discussions, consultations, and adaptation. Generally, it is complex due to the involvement of multiple several stakeholders.

Many evaluations require subject preparation or training. For instance, subjects must be trained for spirometry evaluations. Detailed bowel preparation is required before colonoscopy. Such operational aspects should be considered while developing the protocol.

When third-party laboratories or service providers (central laboratory) are involved in any of the evaluations, the identification, evaluation, and qualification should proceed along with study planning. The lead time for service setup must be factored into planning. Operational challenges should be foreseen and worked out especially while dealing with several third-party service providers. Sites may outsource some laboratory work to other organizations and due diligence by the sites to ensure quality and capability of those organizations is necessary. Validation of equipment at the clinical sites should be considered at an early stage and could be considered part of site selection process. If service providers are used for supplying equipment, validation information should also be collected.

Often, while working with service providers, detailed requirements are overlooked at the initial evaluation stage. It could become troublesome later in the trial after award of the work order. Changing a service provider in the middle of a trial is not so easy. Critical requirements of each evaluation should be identified and documented as it serves the basis for evaluation of service providers.

Patient and physician-reported questionnaires or instruments are utilized for efficacy measurement in several diseases. Copyright, translation and validation requirements should be considered. Data management of such data needs special attention. If electronic patient diaries are used, data transfer process should be evaluated by the data management team.

The method of data capture, reporting, data transfer from laboratories and contract research organizations should be discussed during planning. Similarly, the process of reporting of data collected through instruments supplied by service providers should be clarified. Data management team should also be involved in these discussions. Dry runs before trial initiation are typically useful.

Certain PD effects may reveal the study treatment allocation due to unique effects in blinded studies. The ways to mitigate such issues must be planned and discussed with the stakeholders. Independent study personnel could be an option for data handling.

In some situations, same PD parameters are measured simultaneously by different devices in a trial for specific purposes. For example, ECG may be recorded by Holter and simple ECG machine. BP may be measured through sphygmomanometer and ambulatory BP measuring device. Blood glucose may be measured through a continuous glucose monitoring (CGM) device and glucometer. In the last example, the CGM is not as accurate or reliable as a glucometer; however, it can provide real-time glucose level data, (every 1 or 5 minutes) which can be confirmed by glucometer in case of hypoglycemia.

Safety alerts are often notified to the sponsor or investigators once significant events are identified during data evaluation at central laboratories. It may have important considerations for individual subjects or the overall study conduct. A detailed procedure should be available on the definition of significant events, report format, recipients, turnaround time and blinding considerations.

31. Planning multiple evaluations in a clinical trial

A clinical trial may give an opportunity to evaluate several potential effects of a drug. The nature of evaluations may be pharmacokinetic, clinical, biochemical, pathological, electrophysiological, radiological, patient/physician-reported outcome, pharmacogenomic or proteomic measures. Typically, comprehensive evaluations are part of exploratory trials in early drug development to maximize efforts and gather as much information as possible. In late phase trials, evaluations are more focused when the understanding of the compound is mature, and the objectives of trials are specific to support product registration or therapeutic use.

Each evaluation requires specific subject preparation, prerequisite and logistics to consider. Certain evaluations are simple and quick to perform while others are process or time intensive. Multiple evaluations could create conflicts in managing time, resources or subject preparation while conducting a trial at the site. Meticulous planning is essential at the time of protocol development as well as feasibility evaluation and study set up at the sites.

Here are few points to consider:

- Evaluations should be prioritized based on study objectives.

- Minimizing the number of evaluations keeps the focus of the study.

- Possibility of operational error increases with the number of evaluations.

- Multiple evaluations lead to a complex assessment schedule in the protocol.

- Evaluations should be planned at minimum frequencies to make it less burdensome for the subjects and clinical sites.

- Several study visits may create difficulty in scheduling subject visits in addition to negatively affecting motivation to trial participation.

- Assessment schedules should take into consideration logistics of individual evaluation, subject preparation and training of both subject and site personnel. Wider 'window' periods to perform individual assessments are more practical and reduce deviations.

- When multiple evaluations coincide, the priority sequence should be specified, and appropriate time windows should be provided for each evaluation. For instance, if a blood collection, BP and ECG measurement coincide, it should be specified which one should be done first and which one at the end. The one to be performed last certainly needs a wider window period.

- When several blood samples are planned, the total volume of blood collection should be taken into consideration. There may be ethical concerns especially in certain disease states and children.

- The clinical site should plan resources in terms of staff and infrastructure to handle all the evaluations. In the initial period, the site may minimize enrolment rate to develop familiarity. Mock trials or dry runs may be planned to see that the logistics and staff preparedness is adequate.

- Chances of mix up in samples due to improper labelling should be considered. When several biological samples are to be taken, inadvertent sample collection in wrong tubes is a possibility. Proper planning, training and color coding of sample tubes for easy identification are helpful.

- Protocol deviations should be anticipated while several evaluations are planned. Reportable protocol deviations should be defined in the protocol deviation management plans.

- A domiciled stay could be considered on specific days when there are several assessments to have better control over the situation where possible.

32. Prevention of pregnancy in a clinical trial

Investigational products may have a potential for adverse effect on reproduction. Specific instructions are provided in the protocol for subject selection, contraceptive use during and after the trial as well as follow up requirements after trial completion and in case of pregnancy.

During early drug development period, preclinical studies provide an indication of the potential for such toxicity. Such studies look for an effect on fertility, reproduction, embryo-fetal development, childbirths as well as maternal and child health. It is generally need-based, incremental in nature and planned to supplement the information required for drug development decision making. Information on compounds with similar chemical structure is also taken into consideration.

For a marketed drug, the investigations are expected to be complete to caution the users as necessary. It may be supplemented with human data if a drug is in the market for a long time. Although such data may be available for a new drug, it would be generally limited. The details of evaluations for reproductive toxicity assessment and determination of specific recommendations are outside the scope of this discussion.

Prevention of pregnancy in clinical trials is necessary to avoid any harm to the unborn child, trial participants, or interference in trial assessments. Protocol or the investigator's brochure should include guidance about three groups of population i.e. female study subjects, male study subjects, and female partners of male study subjects. The risk to female partners of male participants arises as drugs secreted in semen may be absorbed from the female reproductive track and thereby gain access to systemic circulation.

Here is the basis for decision making:
- Availability of genotoxicity and reproductive toxicity data
- Availability of any human data

- Type of compound, pharmacology, evidence from other compounds of the same class
- Target population for which the compound is under development
- Study population

Clarity required on the following aspects in the protocol or other appropriate study documents:

- Whether both male and females will participate in the trial
- Whether women of childbearing potential (WOCBP) will participate in the trial
- Definition of women of childbearing potential
- Definition of women of non-childbearing potential (WONCBP)
- Evidence required to demonstrate if female subjects are WONCBP
- Procedure to deal with subjects who are WONCBP due to sexual orientation, lifestyle
- Definition and examples of acceptable contraceptive practice
- Duration of contraceptive practice (e.g. 5 half-life post the last drug administration or duration of replication of a live vaccine)
- Method and frequency of undertaking pregnancy tests for female subjects (all women vs. WOCBP, urine test vs. serum test for pregnancy)
- Contraception requirement for female partners of male subjects
- Follow up plan in case of pregnancy
- Plan for consent, information or follow up in case of female partners of male subjects

The requirement of pregnancy prevention in the trial should be discussed with the subjects. All the relevant information including the potential to cause fetal harm, recommended contraceptive use, duration of contraceptive use and follow up plan in case of pregnancy should be included in the informed consent form (ICF). A separate document for information may be provided to female partners of male subjects with the relevant information.

The importance of pregnancy prevention should be reminded periodically during the trial, and it should be captured in the source documents (e.g. subject files). Pregnancy tests should be performed at appropriate intervals to rule out the occurrence of pregnancy. It is a good practice to have flexible language in the protocol to allow a pregnancy test as necessary during the trial in addition to predefined time points.

Subjects who are WONCBP due to surgical procedures or medical conditions may be asked to furnish documentation supporting it. Such documents may be verified by the monitor or sponsor's representative. The investigator may contact the primary physician of the subject for more information if necessary.

Often, there is controversy around categorizing women as WONCBP. A female subject may not have sexual intercourse due to separation from partner, religious practice or sexual orientation. Certain surgical procedures may not provide 100% protection from pregnancy theoretically (e.g. chances of re-canalization in tubal ligation surgery). In general, abstinence is not an acceptable method of contraception in clinical trials due to high failure rates. Diagnosis of postmenopausal status based on FSH level may be misleading if a subject is on hormone replacement therapy. Such issues should be clarified in the protocol and discussed with the investigators.

The sites should be consulted about the commonly used contraceptive practices in the country or region. For instance, spermicidal gel is not available or used in many places and such a protocol requirement may be troublesome. The ethics committees or health authorities may recommend a higher level of contraception depending on the profile of the investigational drug (e.g. simultaneous double method of contraception). It is difficult to ensure 100% compliance to contraception requirement; nonetheless, compliance can be improved through proper counselling. Flexible language in the protocol could be considered to allow additional contraceptive options on a case by a case basis with necessary approvals (i.e. sponsor and ethics committee).

Contraception is a sensitive topic to discuss with subjects and their parents in pediatric trials. Site personnel should be skilful to discuss sexual history and contraception with pediatric subjects and the discussion could happen separately (i.e. not in presence of their parents). Generally, such information gathered from subjects is not shared with their parents or guardians. The complexities surrounding legal, cultural, and social aspects should be managed appropriately. Contraception is not recommended for subjects who have not initiated sexual activity.

Guidance should be provided on female subjects or female partners of male subjects who become pregnant. Typically, the pregnancy is followed up until childbirth to evaluate any abnormality in the offspring. It may be of longer duration if considered appropriate. A pregnancy reporting form is completed by the investigator with all the relevant information. Follow up reporting forms are completed subsequently.

33. Trial restrictions

As clinical trials explore safety or efficacy of various interventions in human subjects, one major goal is to accurately estimate and attribute any effect of an intervention when it exists. While entry criteria help in choosing the target population, trial restrictions minimize the confounding factors during trial conduct, so that, the observed effect can be attributed to the experimental intervention without bias. In some instances, it could also play an important role to ensure the safety of trial subjects. When several variables can influence an endpoint, it becomes difficult to estimate the true drug effect unless such confounding factors are controlled.

The trial outcome could be influenced by lifestyles of subjects or protocol compliance in a trial. Importantly, noncompliance with trial restrictions may also unduly expose them to risks in the study. However, any overt restrictions, measures or standards followed or applied in a trial may lead to a scenario, which is far from real-life clinical practice and hence, may have limited applicability to routine practice. Restrictions could involve lifestyle measures, dietary intake, and certain prerequisites before an assessment or certain activities to be performed during the trial. It is usually in the form of 'dos' and 'don't dos'.

The scope of trial restrictions includes any measures after screening until study completion or a longer duration if needed depending upon the study population, design and interventions. If a trial restriction applies to a timeframe preceding screening or baseline visit, it could be considered part of entry criteria.

Examples of trial restrictions are (i) no strenuous physical exercise 7 days prior to first dose until 2 weeks after the last dose (ii) no food intake for 10 hours before drug administration until 4 hours after (iii) no prescription medicines for 3 weeks before first dose until 7 days after study completion (iv) No driving of motor vehicles within six hours of drug administration (v) use of highly effective contraceptive from screening until study completion. In example (iii), a subject may be eligible for randomization if there is no such medication history or by avoiding such medication for 3 weeks prospectively to satisfy the criterion.

Restrictions should be explicitly specified in the protocol without ambiguity. It should be scientifically justifiable, operationally feasible and to the minimum extent required. Restrictions could pose operational challenges to recruitment and retention, or lead to protocol deviations. It may be prudent to consider prior experience with such restrictions or obtain feedback from clinical sites.

Restrictions in a trial are informed to the subjects through the informed consent form (ICF). Importance of the restrictions to the study should be discussed with the subjects and their willingness to follow should be assessed. Subjects should be reminded about the restrictions in each visit and compliance to it should be documented. Key restrictions may be captured in the case report form (CRF) for review and analysis.

Compliance to study restrictions could be verified or implemented through laboratory tests (urine cotinine level measurement for smoking), domiciliation for direct supervision (typically done in pharmacokinetics studies), counselling, study visits (direct supervision such as supervised dosing), diary entry or other innovative methods. Clinical history remains the most commonly used method to assess compliance. Restrictions may have direct (more visits, domiciled stay, or laboratory tests) and indirect (discontinuations or recruitment issues) financial implications.

Clinical sites play a critical role in ensuring compliance with restrictions and field monitors have a responsibility to verify the compliance. It is important to understand that most of the information related to restrictions may be documented in the subject file without the need to capture in the CRF. The monitor gets access to all these documents or opportunity to observe few study procedures in real time during onsite visits. Such observations or review requirements are detailed in the monitoring plan, and the monitoring visits are planned accordingly. Any deviations should be discussed with the site and the sponsor, and any remedial steps necessary should be taken. Typically, the deviations are also reported in the monitoring visit report and followed up in subsequent monitoring visits. Besides the monitoring reports, protocol deviations are reported and managed as per the protocol deviation management plan.

Noncompliance with a restriction is a protocol deviation and may adversely affect the study assessments. Not all restrictions may be equally important, and some degree of flexibility may not affect certain outcome measures significantly. Not all deviations may meet reporting requirements (i.e. significant protocol deviations). Instances, which may require subject withdrawal from the trial due to noncompliance, should be clarified in the protocol or any other study document. Alternatively, decisions could be taken on a case by case basis after discussion with the sponsor's medical monitor. Noncompliance with restrictions may have safety concerns in some situations. For instance, if a drug has sedative effects, driving should be prohibited after treatment.

34. Protocol referenced documents

ICH GCP guidance has provided a comprehensive list of topics to be included in a clinical trial protocol. While all the essential information in the protocol as a single document can be helpful, it also takes away the flexibility, as not every detail is available at the time of protocol finalization. Moreover, as the protocol is the basic document that is reviewed by regulatory authorities and ethics committees, any amendment triggers a fresh round of review cycle.

ICH GCP allows some of the information expected in the protocol to be contained in other protocol referenced documents. This approach is commonly adopted to provide key essential information in the protocol while specific details are described in other documents such as investigator's brochure, procedures manual, laboratory manual, pharmacy manual, enrolment plan, clinical site SOP, etc which are referenced although not available at the time of protocol finalization. Typically, these documents are either not required to be submitted to authorities or are only submitted for information.

It is a good practice to stipulate in the protocol that additional information would be provided in certain documents regarding certain topics. For example, it could be mentioned that additional information about an investigational product (IP) handling at the site would be provided in a pharmacy manual. The pharmacy manual typically covers procedures to receive the investigational product, dose preparation, precaution to maintain blinding when necessary, administration, supply/resupply, storage and destruction.

Similarly, additional information about certain trial procedures (e.g. training on home blood glucose measurement, aseptic venipuncture technique, triplicate blood pressure assessment, completion of a patient reported-outcome questionnaire) could be provided in the procedure manual. The laboratory manual typically has details of lab kits, blood sample collection, processing, aliquot preparation, labelling, storage, shipment procedures, sample management at the central laboratory, analysis plan, data management, supply/resupply of kits, contact details of the laboratories, reference ranges, etc.

There are no recommended specific formats for these documents, although organizations may have own templates to cover specific topics with provisions for customization as necessary. It is important to keep such additional documents brief with precise and concise information without any redundancies between different documents. Duplication of information in different documents typically leads to inconsistency and creates dependency when one is amended.

Relevant functions lead the creation and finalization of these documents. Generally, the process is initiated once the protocol is final or in the final draft stage. Relevant members of the trial team review these documents similar to the protocol. Input from clinical sites (or selected sites) is particularly helpful as it contains operational information for sites. It is a good practice to keep these documents in the final draft stage until close to trial initiation to minimize version changes due to last moment amendments.

35.Run-in period

Run-in period between screening and initiation of investigational treatment helps to prepare potential subjects for a clinical trial. Common reasons for the provision of a run-in period in trials are to exclude subjects who are found to be noncompliant, placebo responders, ill-tolerated to treatments, or non-responders. It is often used to withdraw previous treatments, initiate standard of care or obtain stable baseline parameters. Subjects are followed up in one or more subsequent visits with safety and other study assessments to confirm eligibility before randomization. Placebo may be used during a run-in period.

Run-in periods are considered part of the trial and can be only initiated after obtaining consent. Any treatments such as placebo, the standard of care or modification to previous background medication during this period are considered trial interventions. Appropriate monitoring as well as safety and efficacy assessment is typically performed.

Strong scientific basis should exist for the run-in period in a trial taking into consideration study design, disease population, potential adverse events and ethical principles. The risk and benefit of a run-in period should be discussed in the protocol. Here are some scenarios which may be encountered in a trial (i) Patient is stable on a therapy (ii) Patient is on a therapy, however, the response is not satisfactory (iii) Patient is not on any therapy and the disease is not controlled (iv) Patient is not on protocol required background therapy but response is satisfactory (v) Patient is on protocol required drug product but not on the protocol required dose. Some of these scenarios could be complex to handle in the context of a clinical trial.

Run-in period and its relevance to the trial should be clarified in the informed consent form (ICF). Subjects should be explained about this provision during an informed consent process. While assessing placebo response, the placebo administration during the run-in period need not be disclosed to subjects, it is acceptable to mention only that placebo will be administered at some time during the trial. Rescue medication should be planned appropriately during placebo run-in period in disease conditions, especially if treatment withdrawal is needed. Lack of benefit during placebo run-in period and frequent requirement of rescue medication may lead to loss of interest from subjects.

When a modification to a stable treatment regimen is required, patients may become apprehensive about their health and may be reluctant to participate in the trial. Subjects should be provided with detailed information about the rationale and risk involved to make an informed decision. Similar concerns may be raised by the investigators, ethics committees and authorities.

In some studies, close supervision may be required for standardization of diet, lifestyle or background treatment during the run-in period. Domiciling the subjects could be considered and it may affect the overall trial budget and recruitment.

Subject eligibility is assessed during and after the run-in period as per the protocol. In general, repeated multiple evaluations are operationally challenging and cumbersome. For instance, after a month-long run-in period, the subject may fail in vital sign measurement or in a laboratory test due to marginally outside of normal ranges.

36. Case report form

The case report form (CRF) is a commonly used modality to collect subject data from the clinical sites, which are essential for safety and efficacy evaluation of trial interventions. Subject-specific information is recorded in subject files or is available in laboratory reports, which collectively constitute the source document. This information from the source document is reported to the sponsor using the CRF. Certain subject data could be directly transferred to the trial database of the sponsor without the need for CRF entry.

While the source document may contain detailed information about the subject, treatment, disease progress or various evaluations, only essential elements (typically stipulated in the study protocol or another study document) are reported in the CRF. Fundamentally, the data elements that would be statistically analyzed or important for reporting purpose are collected. Certain data is collected only to review protocol compliance. As per the sponsor's process, either data of all subjects who have signed informed consent form or data of only subjects who have been randomized are reported in the CRF.

In confirmatory trials for regulatory purposes, reasons for screen failure are collected. It helps to understand the target population for which the drug approval will be applicable and the profile of the population who were excluded in the trial. This is relevant both for the health authorities and for the sponsors. It is of low relevance in exploratory trials as the objectives are different.

Here are examples of data elements, which may be collected through CRF.

- Identifiers: study number, center number, screening number, randomization number, subject initial, visit number, time, treatment group
- Informed consent: time of informed consent
- Demography: age, sex, height, weight, race, ethnicity
- Medical history: condition, date of diagnosis, condition or problem active at start of study treatment
- Entry criteria: inclusion criteria, exclusion criteria, reasons for screen failure
- Clinical and laboratory assessment: evaluation, result, normal range, clinical significance
- Drug administration record: drug type, dose, unit, time of administration

- Adverse event: event name, start time, end time, severity, seriousness, relationship to study drug, action taken
- Concomitant medication: medication, dose amount, unit, frequency, reason for administration, start time, end time
- Food intake: start time, end time, percentage consumed
- Protocol deviations: description, severity, action taken
- Study completion: completed/discontinued, reason

Traditionally CRF was paper-based, where data is entered with a regular pen in a legible manner. Each CRF page has 2-3 copies apart from the original page that is printed in distinct colors (original in white color, pink and yellow for copies although this is not a regulatory requirement). NCR (No carbon required) papers are utilized for the copies.

Electronic CRF could be web-based or application loaded laptop computer systems. In the latter scenario, the computer systems are transported to clinical sites for data entry. In web-based systems, the CRF can be accessed through the internet from any computer system. In both the modalities, the data is transferred through the internet. Another hybrid modality of digital pen technology is also available. Currently, web-based eCRFs are the norm.

CRF development is initiated along with the protocol development. A draft synopsis or protocol with assessment schedule could be the basis to begin CRF development. Typically, organizations have data collection standard library for simplification and efficiency. A library of data standards or CRF pages makes the process easier for the CRF developer.

For example, data elements for blood pressure (BP) reporting could be if the evaluation was done, subject number, visit number, date, time, position (supine or standing), systolic or diastolic, BP reading and any comments. Some of the options could be pre-specified and need to be only chosen from the available options (for instance supine or standing) while others need to be entered in the blank field (systolic BP value or comments). Electronic formats provide the flexibility of drop-down options, pre-specified values, event-triggered page additions, pre-populated data fields (e.g. subject number, visits number, etc).

Some evaluations in the study may be performed in an unplanned manner due to unforeseen circumstances e.g. a repeat liver function test following abnormality detected during a planned visit. CRF design considers such situations to have provisions for unscheduled visits.

If standard data collection panels are not available, new pages are created or existing pages are customized. It may be called unique or study specific CRF pages. The study team reviews the CRF to confirm that the design is consistent with the protocol and data analysis plan to collect the essential data elements. The CRF is finalized after the protocol is final as it is a protocol dependent document. Certain health authorities and ethics committees require copies of CRF, screenshots of eCRF or paper basis of the eCRF as part of the clinical trial application for review.

The eCRF system is activated after necessary programming. Typically, a user's acceptance test (UAT) is performed by selected study team members before the program is released for use. UAT is an additional step to identify potential gaps. The CRF should be ready and available for data entry at the time of trial initiation.

Infrastructure requirement is minimal for paper CRFs; internet connection and computer systems are required at the sites for eCRFs. Electronic CRF application loaded laptop computers only require internet connection; however, it needs to be transported to the clinical site. The availability of these facilities at the clinical site is evaluated during site selection.

The CRF needs to be modified whenever there is a change to the stipulated data collection (e.g. protocol amendment). It could be cumbersome in terms of timelines and budget depending on the stage of the trial, the extent of modification, and nature of CRF (i.e. paper CRF vs. eCRF).

It is important to ensure the investigator and site staffs are fully aware of the CRF data elements, so that they could document appropriately in the source document or subject file. Typically, elaborate documentation in the source is necessary in the context of clinical trials in comparison to routine clinical practice. For example, physicians only note down key medical history in routine medical practice, while each enquired medical history as required by the protocol must be explicitly recorded in a clinical trial irrespective of its presence status.

The investigator or designated personnel at the clinical site can make CRF entry. Individual login credentials are created for the nominated personnel to access the electronic systems for data entry, so that identity can be traced. During the setup process, site-specific information is collected about the monitor, investigator, and site infrastructure for system configuration. The site personnel should be trained on proper data entry as well as navigation through the electronic system. It is a good practice to demonstrate the site staff on procedures and functions of the electronic system at the site initiation visit or earlier. Typically, helpdesk facility is available to troubleshoot any difficulty.

The field monitors, data management team and other authorized representatives of the sponsor also have access to the database for data review purposes. However, they would have restricted privileges e.g. they cannot enter any data and may not be able to modify any data.

In electronic systems, validation checks are created to prevent inadvertent errors during data entry. There is expected data range for individual assessments, and the system alerts in case of a data, which is outside the programmed range. For instance, if the age ranges as per entry criteria were between 18-55 years, entering a value of 57 would lead to an alert. While programming, expected data ranges are considered in the context of the protocol, study population, laboratory normal range or already present data of a subject. The actual data could be out of range in reality but the system would proactively alert (through a pop-up message once the data is entered or saved) about a potential error depending on the programme. In the context of edit checks with respect to pre-existing data, a significant change to a parameter evaluated in a prior visit could be programmed to raise an alert (e.g. 20% weight difference in two successive visits planned a week apart).

Various scenarios could be programmed to prevent errors through validation checks. A conservative approach with extensive programming creates frequent alerts, while limited validation checks increases the probability of incorrect data entry. Validation checks could be revised if necessary once a significant amount of data entry is complete. Proactive periodic data listing review can minimize the dependence on edit checks. As such, the data management team and trial team review the trial data on an ongoing basis as per data review plans.

In the electronic system, the data seamlessly go to the electronic trial database once entered and saved. In paper CRF, there are two levels of the data transcription (a) from the source document to paper CRF at the clinical site (b) from paper CRF to an electronic trial database by the data management team. At the clinical site, the field monitor reviews the data against the source documents for accurate transcription in a process called source data verification (SDV). At the next level, quality control processes (e.g. double entry of the same data by two operators) ensure correct data entry from paper CRF to an electronic trial database by the data management team.

Any issues in the data (i.e. errors, discrepancies or clarifications) are raised in the form of data queries to the clinical site. Any change or correction to a paper CRF should be dated, initialled, and explained (if necessary) and should not obscure the original entry (i.e. an audit trail should be maintained). Generally, the electronic systems are programmed to maintain the audit trail. Any changes or corrections in CRFs made by data management team must be documented and endorsed by the investigator as per a written procedure. Previously, there were provisions for corrections of obvious errors by the sponsors without going back to the investigators for endorsement. Lists of obvious corrections, which may be made, are notified to the investigators at the beginning of the trial. However, this is no longer in practice universally.

Operationally, paper or computer loaded CRFs are logistically cumbersome. It needs to be physically transported to the clinical site and retrieved. Any modifications can't be readily implemented. Computer loaded CRF systems have to be synchronized with the server after each session of data entry, and incomplete data transfer due to synchronization error is common. Paper CRF has a different set of challenges during query resolution due to the inefficient paper-based system of communication between the data management team and the clinical site staff. However, paper CRF could be cost-effective and efficient for simple and single-center trials.

eCRFs from various service providers are available and some are more user-friendly and offer greater flexibility than others. For example, in blinded trials, there may be a requirement to have restricted access to certain pages of eCRF to only a set of blinded personnel with the site staffs and the data management team. While selecting a vendor, such aspects should be considered.

37.Informed consent form (ICF)

Informed consent is key to ethical research and ICF serves two notable purposes (a) providing essential information about the research (b) contract between the investigator and the research subject on the terms of participation. If the research is planned in a population who are incapable to consent themselves, an acceptable proxy such as a legal guardian or other representative may consent on behalf of a subject. As per the ICH GCP, both the informed consent discussion and the written informed consent form and any other written information to be provided to subjects should include explanations of the following:

- That the trial involves research.

- The purpose of the trial.

- The trial treatment(s) and the probability for random assignment to each treatment.

- The trial procedures to be followed, including all invasive procedures.

- The subject's responsibilities.

- Those aspects of the trial that are experimental.

- The reasonably foreseeable risks or inconveniences to the subject and, when applicable, to an embryo, fetus, or nursing infant.

- The reasonably expected benefits. When there is no intended clinical benefit to the subject, the subject should be made aware of this.

- The alternative procedure(s) or course(s) of treatment that may be available to the subject, and their important potential benefits and risks.

- The compensation and/or treatment available to the subject in the event of trial related injury.

- The anticipated prorated payment, if any, to the subject for participating in the trial.

- The anticipated expenses, if any, to the subject for participating in the trial.

- That the subject's participation in the trial is voluntary and that the subject may refuse to participate or withdraw from the trial, at any time, without penalty or loss of benefits to which the subject is otherwise entitled.

- That the monitor(s), the auditor(s), the IRB/IEC, and the regulatory authority(ies) will be granted direct access to the subject's original medical records for verification of clinical trial procedures and/or data, without violating the confidentiality of the subject, to the extent permitted by the applicable laws and regulations and that, by signing a written informed consent form, the subject or the subject's legally acceptable representative is authorizing such access.

- That records identifying the subject will be kept confidential and, to the extent permitted by the applicable laws and/or regulations, will not be made publicly available. If the results of the trial are published, the subject's identity will remain confidential.

- That the subject or the subject's legally acceptable representative will be informed in a timely manner if information becomes available that may be relevant to the subject's willingness to continue participation in the trial.

- The person(s) to contact for further information regarding the trial and the rights of trial subjects, and whom to contact in the event of trial-related injury.

- The foreseeable circumstances and/or reasons under which the subject's participation in the trial may be terminated.

- The expected duration of the subject's participation in the trial.

- The approximate number of subjects involved in the trial.

- There may be additional local and country-specific requirements which must be included in the ICF. Information on pregnancy avoidance requirement, contraceptive practice as well as follow up plan in case of pregnancy should be carefully and explicitly mentioned.

Operationally, ICF is developed by the investigator in agreement with the sponsor. Alternatively, (typically in multi-centric trial) a model ICF is prepared by the sponsor and provided to the investigators for customization as per local standards and ethics committee guidance. For practical purposes, an English language ICF is developed, and it is translated into local languages as necessary. The accuracy of translation is validated through an independent reviewer or through back translation to English and comparison.

The ICF is expected to be written in a simple and nontechnical language, so that even a layman is able to understand. The ICF is prepared with reference to the protocol, investigator's brochure, approved drug label or any other study related documents. ICF is version controlled, and it is finalized after the protocol, although it could be drafted along with the protocol. The ICF should refer to the latest version of the protocol. Typically, a QC step is performed with a checklist to ensure compliance with GCP requirement.

Trial procedures and most of the other information in the ICF must be consistent with the protocol. When the protocol is amended, or new information is available about the investigational product, the ICF may have to be updated through an amendment. The subjects already enrolled need to be re-consented with the amended ICF in order to make subjects aware of the new information on risk-benefit, study procedures or terms and conditions. New subjects consent with the amended version of ICF directly.

The ICF and the translated versions are approved by the ethics committee and health authorities as per local regulations. The ethics committee may request modifications, which must be implemented through an amendment. The health authority may suggest a modification to the protocol or ICF, which in turn requires CF amendment. Generally, version change is required for a document (protocol, ICF etc), once it has been shared with the ethics committee, health authority or investigators.

Trials may have optional procedures (pharmacogenetic sample collection, biomarker sample collection) in addition to the obligatory study procedures. In such cases, additional ICFs or optional clauses in the main ICF are provisioned which provides information about the additional procedures and seeks participation in the optional procedures along with the main study. Such additional ICFs are used along with the main study ICF and it need not have all the elements discussed above. A subject could refuse the optional procedures and still participate in the trial. In some countries, ICFs may be required for testing sexually transmitted diseases (e.g. HIV).

Often there is scientific desire to store leftover biological samples (i.e. after testing protocol-specified analysis) for future research. Such samples could be very invaluable for research; however, it is also necessary to inform subjects about such use of samples. A specific section may be added to the ICF to clarify the terms of such storage and future analysis. Generally, such provisions are optional, and subjects could indicate their agreement (e.g. use of a checkbox). CRFs are designed to capture such information in order to make this info readily accessible.

38. Investigational drug product in clinical trial

Pharmaceutical industry-sponsored clinical trials usually have investigational drug products (IP) as the intervention. ICH GCP defines IP as "A pharmaceutical form of an active ingredient or placebo being tested or used as a reference in a clinical trial, including a product with a marketing authorization when used or assembled (formulated or packaged) in a way different from the approved form, or when used for an unapproved indication, or when used to gain further information about an approved use."

As the definition goes, an IP can be an active drug, placebo or active comparator, a marketed product or one under investigation. The IP is sensitive from a regulatory and legal perspective and is subjected to rules and regulations of individual countries or states. IP needs to be manufactured, packaged, labelled, transported, stored, dispensed, used and destroyed in appropriate conditions as per regulations. It needs to be handled by authorized personnel, and its accountability must be maintained at all times. Any deviation may violate applicable regulations or potentially alter safety and efficacy outcome in clinical trials.

IP supply can be a complex affair depending on the study design, scale of clinical trial and countries involved. Meticulous planning is the norm and is usually managed by a specialized function.

Here are few scenarios for discussion, but it could be quite different in real life.

- IP supplied by the sponsor to the clinical site as bulk supply in an open label, single treatment arm trial. The IP is prepared into individual packs based on the subject number at the clinical site.

- IP supplied as patient packs by the sponsor to the clinical site in an open label, single treatment arm trial. IP is dispensed as per subject number at the clinical site.

- IP supplied by the sponsor to the clinical site as bulk supply in an open label, randomized, multiple treatment arm trial. The IP is prepared into individual packs based on the subject number and randomization list or treatment allocation cards at the clinical site.

- IP supplied by sponsor to the clinical site as bulk supply in a blinded, randomized trial with multiple treatment arms. The IP is prepared into individual packs based on the subject number and randomization list or treatment allocation cards by an independent (unblinded) pharmacist. However, the subject, investigator and other clinical site staff remain blinded to treatment allocation.

- IP supplied by a sponsor to the clinical site as patient packs in a blinded, randomized trial with multiple treatment arms. IP is dispensed as per subject number and randomization list or treatment allocation cards.

Randomization or treatment allocation is closely linked to IP supply in a randomized study. The randomization list could be supplied to the trial site either for all subjects or on demand where the subject number and treatment allocation are provided once the site has an eligible subject. An 'on demand' process is typically required for a study with multiple clinical sites, and it is typically managed through interactive response technologies (IRT).

IP handling is regulated, and permissions are required to pass borders of countries or states. In the setting of a clinical trial, such permissions are subject to the approval of the trial in a country. Several documents on quality, manufacturing, composition, pharmacology, assay, and stability about the IP are required for permission of a clinical trial. A drug product, which is approved for marketing in one country, may not have approved status in another country. Even, an approved drug product can only be used in a clinical trial after necessary permissions. IP may have different names for one compound depending on the stage of development, formulation or country of origin. IP label typically has the trial codename for identification.

IP supply is a multifunctional team effort led by IP supply function. Several persons are involved in planning, manufacturing, testing, packaging, labelling, documentation and shipment. IP supply is a key limiting step for a clinical trial initiation and it should be considered well in advance taking into consideration the lead time of each of the steps. Due to the number of steps and documentation requirements, close coordination is crucial until the arrival of IP at the clinical site pharmacy.

In the early phases of drug development, the manufacturing process is not well established and small quantities of IP are manufactured to meet the clinical trial requirement. As such, only a few trials of limited sample size are conducted in the early phase of drug development. Formulation research progresses along with clinical drug development. In late phases of development or in the post-approval period, availability of adequate IP may not be an issue once the final market formulation is established. IP is manufactured in batches of a prescribed size having a definite period of shelf life for its use and each batch must pass certain quality standards before release for use.

Once a high-level overview or concept of the trial is available, IP requirement is evaluated. Overages and potential changes to the study design (duration, sample size or dose) should be taken into consideration. If the trial has active or placebo control arms in a blinded design, additional consideration is required for matching the appearance of treatments. Typically, modification to the active pills may be cumbersome and time-consuming, although possible by certain methods such as over encapsulation. It is generally not difficult to manufacture or buy placebo that looks similar to the active drugs.

Blinding is easier to enforce at the clinical site once matching placebo is available. Here is an example for understanding. For a three-arm design (Two active comparators and placebo), each subject has to take two pills for effective blinding (i) comparator 1 + placebo for comparator 2 (ii) placebo for comparator 1 + comparator 2 (iii) placebo for both comparator 1 and 2. If the dosing schedules for the comparators are different, it could be managed by use of matching placebo. Blinding for drugs with a parenteral route of administration could be similarly planned.

When drug products are purchased from the market for use in trials, approval status in the target countries and documentation requirement for trial application should be evaluated. It may not be always possible to get appropriate documentation to support the use of the comparators in a country, where the drug product is not approved. If necessary, clinical sites can directly purchase marketed medications (as per protocol) for a trial and the expenses are reimbursed by the sponsor. There may be a need for analysis of these drug products to generate the certificate of analysis (CoA) to confirm quality. Specialized laboratories are available to conduct the tests for CoA if it cannot be obtained from the manufacturer.

The study design (blinding requirements, comparator drugs, randomization, drug preparation or need for placebo) should be discussed with the IP supply group for feasibility. Feedback from regulatory affairs group is helpful to understand the regulatory requirement regarding the IP in different countries where the trial is envisaged. Such discussions should take place early in the planning stage.

The IP and the treatment plan are described in the protocol. The description about the IP includes the drug product, identification, general handling, storage, dispensing, retrieval, destruction, retention, and accountability. The aspects about treatment plan include treatment arms, treatment allocation, blinding, dosage regimen, drug administration, any dose adjustment, discontinuation criteria, concomitant medications, prohibited treatments, rescue medications, compliance criteria and method for checking compliance. If the preparation and administration procedure of IP at the clinical site is complex, it should be detailed in a separate IP manual. Details of IP handling are typically not necessary to be described in the protocol. Instructive videos may be helpful to demonstrate the steps.

The entire process of drug handling, storage condition, monitoring of storage condition and administration procedure should be discussed with the clinical site from a feasibility perspective at the time of site selection. Documentation related to drug handling is critical in clinical trials. It is generally supervised to some extent by the field monitor (both real-time and retrospective) for compliance with the protocol or other instructions. The extent of such monitoring requirements should be specified in the monitoring plan.

IP may be supplied to a clinical site as a bulk supply or subject packs. In case of bulk supply, subject-specific packs are prepared at the clinical site by the pharmacist or other authorized study personnel. If the study requires blinding, independent pharmacists need to be involved in preparation and treatment group allocation. Similarly, an independent study monitor is required to monitor such procedure and is not involved in the monitoring of any other study activities.

When repackaging, reconstitution or preparation steps are required for the IP at the clinical site, country-specific regulations need to be followed. Feedback from drug regulatory affairs or clinical site should be taken about it. For instance, in some countries, any packaging or drug reconstitution procedure must be performed in GMP conditions even at the site pharmacy. Similarly, labelling of the IP after repackaging or subject specific packaging should be as per local regulations. All such aspects have to be considered at the time of trial planning.

In bioequivalence trials, 'retention sample' needs to be maintained at the trial site or any other independent facility for potential future evaluation. The quantity of retention sample and the duration of storage requirement may be different for different countries. Typically, a conservative approach is followed to cover different requirements. Sites should have the facility for such long duration storage and it must be evaluated as part of site selection.

39.Protocol review

A protocol is the most important document that describes the fundamental outline to conduct a clinical trial. It is developed by a cross-functional trial team of subject matter experts. Before finalization, the protocol goes through an iterative process of review from scientific, operation, regulatory and ethical perspectives. It ensures that the protocol would not only be feasible but also would achieve the trial objectives.

Organizations typically have internal processes of protocol approval before it can be finalized and shared externally. It must be approved by health authorities and ethics committees as per local regulations before implementation. The review and approval process could be iterative, and it may be quite time-consuming. Any substantial amendment needs to go through fresh approval process. Hence, a modification to the trial protocol as and when required is not a practical option.

It is desirable that all the stakeholders are thoroughly consulted during trial planning to have a protocol that is simple, concise, unambiguous and implementable. Due to the involvement of several people, ambiguity in interpretation is common, and it should be addressed during review by the stakeholders.

Review of the protocol by the drug supply group is important for planning and feasibility of drug supply. Data management is another important group who should review the protocol to ensure accurate data collection. Regulatory affairs group brings important insights about the trial feasibility, approval timelines, and documentation requirement in specific countries. In some cases, health authorities are consulted for feedback on the study design to avoid future questions, rejections, or major design change recommendations.

Often, the protocol is reviewed by external consultants or key opinion leaders (KOL) to ensure external acceptability. All possible stakeholders who are not authoring the protocol should be involved in the review process before finalization. There is usually an internal scientific committee within the organization for review and approval. Typically, a synopsis, concept sheet or a draft protocol is the basis for initial review and discussion. Upper management commitment for the trial should be obtained before discussion with external stakeholders.

Protocol development is an iterative process and dependent on many factors including cost and changing competitive environment. This entire process is driven by the study manager with the support of the clinical trial team.

Investigator(s) play the most important role in the operational success of a trial. Hence, when feasible, protocol and study operational plan should be discussed with the investigators, especially on entry criteria, study restrictions, laboratory ranges, background therapy, dose adjustments, concomitant medications, discontinuation criteria, recruitment challenges, ways to improve recruitment, potential questions from ethics committees and any competing trial at their site. In a large multi-country, multi-center trial, such review by all investigators is not possible and may be fraught with conflicting opinions. In larger trials, a protocol could be developed in consultation with a group of KOLs or co-ordinating investigators representing different regions where the trial is planned.

A clear process for protocol development and review is essential. Protocol review, management of feedback and implementation of modification requests could be complicated sometimes and can be time-consuming and frustrating. The review by different stakeholders can be run in series or in parallel depending on the situation and availability of stakeholders. Sometimes, there could be a few outstanding issues, where decision making is not straightforward. It may be strategic in nature or may have significant financial implications.

Resource planning and budget estimation progress along with protocol development. Different functions should be consulted for cost estimation of activities under their purview in addition to protocol review. Services that would be outsourced need to be identified timely, so that, bidding process can be swiftly initiated once the synopsis or protocol is firmed up.

40. Trial document translation

Trial documents are translated to local languages for health authorities, ethics committees, investigators or trial subjects in countries where English is not the primary language of communication (or if the original documents are in another language). It could be required for investigational product related documents, informed consent form (ICF), protocol, patient or physician-reported outcome scale, patient diary, advertisement, lab manual, etc.

The extent of documentation, which needs to be translated, varies across geographic regions. For instance, in Japan and China, all trial related documents are required in local languages for health authority and ethics committee review; in India, fewer documents such as ICF or subject diary need to be translated for trial subjects, who may not understand English. Routine communications to investigators or health authorities may require translation during trial conduct.

The translation must be done by qualified translators with knowledge of both the languages. The translators may have accreditation by the government or private agencies. Else, their educational qualification may have to be assessed for suitability. The translated version should be certified by the translator for correctness. Copies of CV, certificates of qualification and certificate of translation are generally required for archival.

The translations have to be validated for accuracy. In the validation process, both the documents are matched by another person appropriately qualified in both languages. A similar set of documentation is required for the validation as for the translation (i.e. CV, certificates of qualification and certificate of validation). Validation could also be done by back translation of the translated document to the original language. Subsequently, an independent person matches the translated version to the original English copy.

The need for validation of translations and its documentation as described above may be different for different documents and should be taken into consideration. For instance, weekly newsletters may require lesser stringency than an informed consent form.

Translation of documents may take significant time and resource depending upon the documents to be translated, country or language, and it should be factored into operational planning. Certain translated versions of documents such as ICF or subject advertisement need to be reviewed and approved by an ethics committee before use.

Few terminologies, which do not have appropriate words in the target language, may remain as such with explanations. Date or version number of the documents may also remain as such in the original language if acceptable as per local regulations.

Translated copies (to other languages) should have version control and refer to the original language documents (name, version and release date). The translated copies may follow a separate version control. For instance, an English ICF may have version 3 whereas the translated version may have version 2 if one of the versions was not translated.

41.Financial planning in clinical trial

A significant portion of drug development cost is spent on clinical trials. For each drug development program, the budget is estimated for all foreseen clinical trials as per the clinical development plan and it is updated periodically when the development plan is revised. Budget is estimated for all development programs similarly at an organization level. R&D expenditure is allocated on a yearly and multi-year basis and is further broken down for each program depending on priority. In certain countries, there are tax incentives on the R&D expenditure that organizations like to gain.

Yearly expenditure for each program is estimated considering the planned and ongoing trials, while the budget for each trial is estimated based on projected expenditure or actual budget of that trial. Yearly expenditure is projected for trials planned to run over multiple years and quarterly break up may be required for better planning. Budget and resource allocation process may widely vary depending on the size of the organization, nature of research and business model.

While estimating budget for an individual trial, the entire trial activity is broken down to various sub-activities such as clinical work, monitoring, data management, central laboratory work, bio-analytical work, site identification, and so on. These sub-activities are usually further broken up into specific work terms (typically called line items). Cost of conducting each sub-activity is estimated taking feedback from the respective functions. It is important to identify the specific activities, which would be outsourced; some organizations predominantly depend on internal resources, whereas others largely depend on outsourcing. Budget estimation is more precise once actual bids or feedbacks are available from service providers or responsible functions.

Increasingly, an initial budget is estimated utilizing available online tools such as GrantPlan, ClearTrials, Grants Manager (Medidata) or salary.com. Such websites provide access to the database of negotiated procedure cost in clinical trials across therapeutic areas in different regions or countries obtained from various CROs or sponsors. Such tools help to determine the appropriate cost of trial procedures or salary information of the personnel conducting a trial. Similarly, cost of various services such as data management, monitoring or biostatistics can also be estimated.

It is important to understand the concept of Fair Market Value (FMV) in the context of clinical trials. One of the definitions is the price at which bona fide sales have been consummated for assets of like type, quality, and quantity in a particular market at the time of acquisition. There is a considerable difference in opinion how such data should be interpreted as there could be variation attributed to a specific situation of a trial. Generally, organizations have internal procedures on use of such tools and budget approval. Any granted fee above FMV is scrutinized because it could be construed as attempts to influence an investigator.

Trial design has direct implication on the budget. Any major change to the study design may significantly change the scope of work and hence, the budget. Sometimes, trial design is revised based on the cost factor. Once the design is firmed up and no significant change to the budget is anticipated, management approval could be obtained. Internal budget approval processes vary in different organizations.

123

While working with service providers, trial work should be awarded only after securing internal budget approval. Generally, trial-related activities could begin only after contract execution unless it is as per the master service agreement or usual business practice. Cancelling a trial after award of work or contract execution may attract a penalty, as it would have triggered activities by the service providers. Generally, contracts have specific clauses to handle such situations.

It is important to understand the standard unit costs of a particular service. Examples of units are per hour (medical writing), per visit (monitoring) or per table/graph (statistical analysis). It helps to prevent any undue cost escalation by the service providers in the middle of a trial when the scope of work changes. It is possible to obtain bids for multiple scenarios if potential additional services are foreseen or contemplated. There is no opportunity for competitive bidding once a service provider has been selected. Changing a service provider in the middle of a trial is usually not an easy option.

Trial budget expenditure should be reviewed periodically. Any significant budget increase during the trial poses a unique challenge, and it should be anticipated from a risk management perspective. Usual reasons include poor recruitment, additional sites, delays, or significant design change. Organizations usually have operative limits to accommodate any cost escalation. Once the limit is exceeded, fresh budget approval from the management is required. For trials spanning multiple years, budget allocation for each financial year is taken into account. Schedule of payment to service providers and total planned expenditure per year are important considerations.

Service providers should be advised to raise invoices in a timely manner to meet the expenditure target if the services have been rendered. Whenever there is any change to the yearly planned expenditure, necessary adjustment is required as per standard accounting practices.

42.Clinical site identification and selection

Clinical sites recruit and manage the subjects in a clinical trial and play the major role in the operational success of a trial. Adequately equipped and experienced clinical trial site with the necessary infrastructure and trained manpower is required to safeguard the trial subjects and generate high-quality data to support the trial objectives. Broadly, there are two types of clinical sites i.e. clinical pharmacology units (CPU) or hospitals. CPUs are specialized facilities to handle trials in healthy human subjects, whereas, trials in patients are conducted in hospitals or its outpatient facilities. This categorization is a bit arbitrary and broad though.

Clinical sites may be also categorized depending on their primary interest and the subject population they handle. Typically, specialized organizations cater to healthy subject trials and the primary business of such organizations is clinical trial conduct. In comparison, the primary business of hospitals or academic centers (with attached hospitals), where patient trials are conducted, is patient care while clinical trial conduct is of secondary interest. Sometimes, a third category may exist i.e. research facilities in selected disease conditions where trials and patient care get equal priority. Generally, such facilities handle chronic disease conditions such as COPD, hypertension, asthma, diabetes, arthritis, neuropathy, neurological diseases, etc. Clinical pharmacology studies in specific patient populations (e.g. hepatic or renal failure) could be conducted at such centers.

Centers dealing with healthy subjects generally have good infrastructure, trained manpower, adequate staff, access to laboratories and equipment. The criteria for site selection for such sites is focused on quality, cost, timelines, regulatory environment, previous regulatory inspections of the facilities, experience, and reputation. Recruitment is typically not a concern. On the other hand, all aspects need to be considered in case of centers handling patient trials, as many sites may not fulfil the basic expectations.

Sponsors or contract research organizations (CRO) conducting clinical trials maintain a database of potential clinical sites and investigators. This is an ongoing activity, and the information about the sites or investigators is periodically updated. It may be possible to generate a report in the desired format from such databases (e.g. trial sites for diabetes in India). There are also proprietary databases from service providers, who gather information about trial sites from publically available (ClinicalTrials.gov, regional registries) sources or other sources.

Such databases are useful to obtain preliminary information about potential sites (e.g. areas of specialization, available disease populations, data on previous trials, prior audits/inspections, enrolment rate, conflicting trials, potential issues, infrastructure and ethics committee function). With a bit of research, potential investigators could be shortlisted for further evaluation. Site selection and recruitment strategy take into consideration trial complexity, design, patient population, sample size, potential countries, recruitment target for individual countries, investigators' profile, prior experience, etc. A draft synopsis or protocol may be the basis for initiating site identification and evaluation.

A site selection questionnaire or checklist is prepared to capture specific requirements of a trial protocol in addition to general requirements of trial conduct. It should cover aspects such as investigator's experience, prior experience of the site, availability of patients, manpower, research equipment, infrastructure, awareness of GCP, availability of SOPs on key procedures, prior audit or inspection, ethics committee, access to laboratory or other diagnostic facility, accreditation, standard of care, trial awareness in the locality, discontinuation rates in previous similar trials, logistics, and so on. From a practical perspective, it is important to identify the critical requirements of a trial and such issues should be discussed first. Typically, this checklist could be of several pages depending on the trial.

Site selection is a sequential process and begins with identification of potential sites from databases or prior experience. Generally, sponsors prefer clinical sites where they have prior experience and familiarity. Trial sites with a history of inspection by regulatory authorities without any major findings are highly preferred. The usual sequence is to obtain initial feedback through the checklist and then follow it with detailed telephonic discussion and in-person site visit. While planning a site selection visit, preliminary information about the prospective site helps in an effective discussion. Critical elements should be discussed upfront with the site coordinator or the investigator.

A site evaluation visit broadly comprises of an introduction with the site staff, facility tour, review of site working processes or SOPs, review of qualification and training of site personnel and discussion of protocol specific elements. The site staff may be asked to explain the workflow of trial activities from recruitment to end of a trial. Processes of recruitment, informed consent, pharmacy, drug administration, study evaluations, laboratory work, document archive and training records of site staff are typically reviewed in detail. Critical equipment should be checked for working condition, backup plan, validation, and availability hours. Availability of internet and computers are no longer a concern these days from a data management perspective at most sites.

Protocol specific elements such as entry criteria, study restriction, follow-up requirements, drug storage, laboratory assessment, adverse event management, the standard of care and other trial specific logistic issues should be discussed. Site selection process also gives an opportunity to assess trial feasibility in general. This may be an opportunity to adjust protocol elements to improve feasibility based on feedback received from the potential sites.

Financial aspects such as investigator's fee, hospitalization cost, laboratory fee, any overhead expenses, ethics committee fee and mode of payment should be discussed with the site. Contract and invoice management processes should be clarified. Any specific regulations governing trials at the site should be discussed and clarified.

Besides the objective assessment, many subjective aspects are also important. For instance, interest and attitude of the investigator and site staff are important considerations for trial success. Uncooperative and apparently busy investigators may turn out to be key barriers to effective trial conduct. Workload, holiday schedule, staff turnover, mode of employment of staff (full-time or part-time), site quality assurance processes are important considerations.

Many of the deficiencies or concerns identified during site evaluation are discussed with the site for a possibility of improvement. Sites may promise to address the deficiencies and it could be re-evaluated later on the progress. Some of those sites could be considered as backup options.

A site selection report is prepared for each site with the final decision and is archived in the trial master file. Often, site identification and selection activity are outsourced to CROs. However, it should be closely supervised by the sponsor.

43.Outsourcing in clinical trial

The pharmaceutical, biotechnology, and medical device companies discover, develop, manufacture and sell healthcare products and are the usual organizations who conduct industry-sponsored clinical trials. They may have own R&D functions to carry out the research work; however, many of the activities may not be conducted in-house due to lack of resources. Often, the business model is to focus on core areas for better returns on resource investment, while services can be availed on demand from the market for activities, which are standardized and easily available. Sponsor organizations contract out such activities to external business partners in a process called 'outsourcing'.

In the last two decades, many contract research organizations (CRO) have emerged that offer various services in clinical research. Some of the CROs offer specific specialized services. For instance, certain CROs specialize in laboratory services, electrophysiology evaluations, logistics, site management, monitoring, and so on. Increasingly, there is a trend of sponsors minimizing dependence on own R&D infrastructure while expanding reliance on outsourcing which is perceived as cost-effective.

The first step in the outsourcing process is the identification of the scope of work. Typically, a document is prepared with details of the scope of work including timelines and any specific requirements. It is the basis for the invitation of bids or discussion with external service providers (i.e. request for proposal). The study protocol or synopsis is usually shared with the service providers so that they have a better understanding of the requirement. A confidentiality agreement must be in place before sharing trial documents with external partners.

The potential external partners provide their feasibility evaluation, cost estimate and any concern about the services in a proposal. Often, there are discussions to ensure that the expectations are well understood. Sponsors typically negotiate to get a better price or favorable timelines before awarding the work. Quality, expertise, experience, cost and working relationship are the usual considerations while selecting a service provider. Comparison of cost from different service providers could be tricky; hence, cost break up is usually obtained in a common format. Sponsors typically have a list of 'preferred partners' for specific activities based on prior evaluations and experience.

The sponsor has the responsibility to perform due diligence while outsourcing trial activities. The working processes of service providers are reviewed by subject matter experts and quality assurance representatives. At times, the external partners may be asked to follow a set of sponsor's SOPs and work processes.

Prior to initiation of any trial activity, a contract is executed with the service provider. However, it may not be the case all the time, and certain preparatory work could be started depending on the business model and industry practice. Sponsors may also have master service agreements with certain service providers to initiate some activities once the task is awarded. This should be evaluated from a regulatory perspective, as certain activities should not be initiated without a valid contract. For instance, enrolment at the clinical site should not be initiated before contract execution.

Operational aspects of outsourcing are usually managed by the outsourcing function of the sponsor. The business development function is the counterpart at the service provider's organization to manage the operational aspects. The process of outsourcing should be initiated sufficiently in advance keeping in mind the time required for inviting bids, evaluation, contracts, preparatory activities and lead time for setup.

Sometimes, the study design is reworked based on the initial budget estimate and feasibility feedback. During the trial, any change to the scope of work is implemented through a change order or contract amendment, which may also involve a change in the budget. The organizational policy may vary, and it should be followed for outsourcing activities.

The milestones and quality of the deliverable are monitored periodically as per contract by sponsor's project managers or subject matter experts. Even when an activity is outsourced, the ultimate responsibility remains with the sponsor. It is important to forge a good working relationship with the associates of the service providers. Every effort should be made to foster an environment of one team with mutual trust and respect. The expectations should be consistent with the scope of work in the contract.

An escalation procedure is typically available, and it should be solicited when necessary in a professional manner using the right channel. After completion of the work, any outstanding issues should be resolved and documented. The service providers are generally assessed in terms of quality, proficiency, and lessons learned for future work.

It is important to understand the processes of the service providers to manage requests for bids, work orders, change orders or contract modifications. Personnel at the CROs are required by their organizations to follow internal processes to manage such requests from sponsors.

Broadly there are three different models how sponsors work with their vendor partners. The traditional way of working is trial by trial outsourcing model. Vendors are selected for each new trial through competitive bidding. The challenge in this model is managing too many vendors, processes, new people and their training requirement and it has an inherent propensity to bring down efficiency.

With the objective to improve efficiency, another modality is a preferred partner model. A set of trials or related activities are outsourced to a limited set of organizations. Often, all or a set of trials in a program or multiple programs are outsourced to one vendor to improve efficiency. Sponsors and their contracted organizations work out governance structures for operational modalities, performance monitoring, and escalation resolution. Contracted organizations are expected to show more commitment, align internal processes, require lesser training and offer better pricing in return for higher volume of work.

A newer concept of virtual clinical organization model is gaining traction to manage R&D uncertainty through greater transparency, close cooperation, strategic alignment, and risk sharing. Managing manpower is a constant challenge for any sponsor organization with peak and trough workloads. The contracted organizations can offer greater flexibility to accommodate resources through redistribution as they work with multiple sponsors. In this model, sponsors align with the vendor organizations for a long-term partnership providing insights about product development strategies and resource requirements over several years. Both the organizations streamline business and operational processes for seamless work in an integrated model.

Early engagement with the sponsors is an opportunity to provide key operational insights for better planning. Vendor organizations may also share some of the risks for accountability as sponsors may take strategic decisions as per their advice.

44.Ethics committee

Institutional Review Board or IRB (ICH GCP definition): An independent body constituted of medical, scientific, and non-scientific members, whose responsibility is to ensure the protection of the rights, safety and well-being of human subjects involved in a trial by, among other things, reviewing, approving, and providing continuing review of trial protocol and amendments and of the methods and material to be used in obtaining and documenting informed consent of the trial subjects.

Independent Ethics Committee or IEC (ICH GCP definition):An independent body (a review board or a committee, institutional, regional, national, or supranational), constituted of medical professionals and non-medical members, whose responsibility it is to ensure the protection of the rights, safety and well-being of human subjects involved in a trial and to provide public assurance of that protection, by, among other things, reviewing and approving / providing favorable opinion on, the trial protocol, the suitability of the investigator(s), facilities, and the methods and material to be used in obtaining and documenting informed consent of the trial subjects. The legal status, composition, function, operations and regulatory requirements pertaining to independent ethics committees may differ among countries, but should allow the independent ethics committee to act in agreement with GCP as described in this guideline.

In addition to ICH GCP, local health authorities or other government bodies may lay down principles for the composition and function of IRBs or ethics committees (EC). IRBs/ECs must follow local regulations with respect to its operation. In certain countries, there may be a requirement for registration or accreditation of ECs by health authorities (e.g. in India) to function. ECs should have standard operating procedures on its composition and functioning. These documents may be required for the trial master file.

Ethics committee approvals are mandatory before conducting a clinical trial at a site. In case, the site doesn't have an IRB, approval may be obtained from an independent or central ethics committee, who agrees to review and oversee the trial conduct. IRB and health authority (HA) review may proceed as parallel activities wherever feasible. In some countries, IRB approval is a prerequisite for clinical trial application to HA.

Here are a few tricky situations, which may be encountered in trial operation. Can an investigator approach an independent EC in a situation where the institution has its own IRB? Can a second EC be approached in case there is an unfavorable opinion from one EC? In general, such situations should be avoided. The IRB of the institution should be approached in the former situation and the opinion of the first EC should be respected in the later situation. However, a second EC can be approached if an EC supervising a trial abdicates its responsibility due to administrative reasons (e.g. EC stops functioning).

Ethics committee review, approval, and supervision are a continuous process (from time of application until trial end) and the responsibility doesn't end with the trial approval. Typical documents which are reviewed for trial approval are the protocol, investigator's brochure, informed consent form (ICF), investigators' CV, facility report, source document templates, case report form, advertisements, drug label, translated copies of the documents (if applicable) and trial insurance certificate. Nonetheless, there may be a variation to it as per local guidance or practice. Any amendment to these study documents must be submitted to IRB for approval or as notification before use.

Requirements, procedures, and timelines of the IRB should be considered in trial planning. Usually, the investigator or an investigator's representative is the link between the sponsor and the IRB. It is the investigator's responsibility to obtain necessary trial approvals or address any questions from the IRB in consultation with the sponsor. At times, the sponsor's representative may be invited to the EC /IRB meeting to present the trial protocol or clarify any specific points on the trial interventions. Usually, the sponsor doesn't communicate directly with IRB. However, in an extreme situation of trial misconduct at a site, the sponsor may directly get in touch with the IRB requesting to intervene if the investigator is uncooperative.

The IRB approval should have information about the documents reviewed as well as members who reviewed and voted. The opinion may be favorable, unfavorable, conditional approval subject to modification or request for clarification. Local regulations must be adhered to regarding the format of approval document. Generally, a membership list, the quorum, list of documents reviewed and opinion of the IRB along with any comments/questions are necessary. IRBs may offer an expedited review, which may be necessary for emergencies or meeting timelines.

The IRB is periodically updated on trial progress and on any new information about the trial, especially any new safety data. It includes protocol deviations, changes to the trial facility or investigator, GCP issues, decision by other health authorities or IRBs (if applicable and required), any significant safety data on the investigational product or safety issues in the trial. The study report once available is submitted to IRB at the end of trial. IRB approval may be valid for a certain duration and need to be renewed periodically, it should be considered in long duration trials.

Any decision taken by the sponsor on trial conduct such as trial termination or suspension should be notified to the IRB. Information about study progress such as enrolment, study completion or site closeout should be informed periodically. IRB holds the authority to terminate, suspend or suggest modification (e.g. changes to the ICF, additional laboratory tests to be done at specific visits for safety, etc) to the study proposal at any time to safeguard the trial subjects. Trial subjects can reach out to the IRB to clarify any concern related to the trial. Contact details of the IRB are typically included in the ICF.

IRB fee is paid by the investigator and it is reimbursed by the sponsor. IRB compensation is both for review of proposal and supervision of trial conduct. IRB may charge on a monthly basis for the duration of a trial.

45. Regulatory authority (health or competent authority)

The ICH GCP defines regulatory authorities as 'bodies having the power to regulate'. In the ICH GCP guideline, the expression regulatory authorities include the authorities that review submitted clinical data and those that conduct inspections. These bodies are sometimes referred to as competent authorities.' The terms 'health authority', 'drug agency' or 'regulatory agency' are synonymous with regulatory authority.

These authorities are specific to individual countries and take the decision on drug development, evaluation of drug dossiers and marketing authorization. Regarding clinical trials on pharmaceutical products, health authority (HA) is responsible to evaluate, permit, terminate, suspend and inspect clinical trial conduct in a country. HA of one country may inspect a trial in another country if the data for marketing authorization has origins from that country.

The scope of health authority is twofold with respect to clinical development and clinical trials (i) data requirement for new drug evaluation and marketing authorization (ii) permissions to conduct clinical trials and operational standards. Here are two scenarios as examples.

A. The drug is under development for the UK and a clinical trial to support that is planned in India. The nature of data to be generated from the trial is decided by the UK authority. However, Indian authority decides whether the trial can be conducted in India and the operational standards of trial conduct. Both the authorities can inspect the trial conduct, although the Indian authority has more operational control as it is conducted in India.

B. The drug is under development for the UK and a clinical trial to support that is planned in the UK. Both the aspects (i and ii) are decided by the UK authority.

The HAs lay down guidelines or directives for the extent of data to be generated for a drug approval as well as the way clinical trial should be conducted. Such information is available in public domain for reference (e.g. ICH, EMEA, US FDA, CDSCO websites). Additionally, there is provision to both formally and informally discuss and take feedback on specific drug development programs i.e. the extent and nature of data to be generated for a particular drug under development.

It is a common practice to hold such meetings at important stages of product development for guidance. Such meetings help the sponsor to get clarity on a range of studies needed for evaluation and marketing authorization of a new drug. These are especially useful in situations where there is lack of clarity in certain indications, or when an entirely new class of compound is under development.

Similarly, while planning to conduct a trial, feedback on a trial design may be obtained from HAs of countries where the trial is planned. It helps to optimize resources and timelines by adapting the protocol before formal trial application or alternatively, excluding those countries from consideration where approvals may be difficult to obtain.

It is the responsibility of the sponsor to obtain all necessary permissions from the concerned HA for a trial conduct. The investigator doesn't communicate with the HAs. Regulatory department of the sponsor typically liaises with the HAs. Communication and document submissions are increasingly electronic in nature. Formal face to face meetings or teleconferences/videoconferences are other modalities to discuss with officials of HAs as per local practice.

While planning a trial, country-specific requirement, the procedure of trial application as well as timeline should be understood. For instance, an IND is filed for any new drug investigation in the US and there is a waiting period of 30 days before the first trial could commence. Subsequent trials may be initiated immediately after submitting the trial protocol (and few other documents). In Europe, India and many other countries, trial-specific applications are made, and trials can be initiated only after obtaining approval. In Australia, the HA is only notified about the trials and only IRB approval is the prerequisite to initiate a trial; however, HA may intervene at any point. In certain countries such as China and Japan, all trial documents need to be submitted in the local language.

HAs may approve the trial application, raise questions for clarification, suggest modifications or approve the protocol with suggested changes. In certain countries, it may be required to present the trial protocol to a panel of experts in a face to face meeting and directly resolve any queries. In India, approvals obtained from other reference countries may be provided as supporting information to facilitate approval.

HA is notified periodically of trial progress and any significant new information on the trial, especially safety data with the investigational product (IP). The extent of notifications, its timeline and procedures should be understood from the regulatory functions. Depending on the country, any substantial amendment to the protocol has to be approved by the HA before implementation. Definition of the substantial amendment is available in the guidelines. HA may be notified of start and end of a trial, SAEs in the trial or any other trials involving the concerned IP. Once the trial is completed, the study report is also submitted to HA.

HAs can inspect any trial-related activity (clinical conduct, laboratory analysis, data management, etc) at any location to verify that the trial conduct is as per regulations, SOPs and ethical principles. All organizations (e.g. sponsor, investigator) involved in clinical trials are obliged to co-operate in inspection, which can be pre-planned, or unannounced. Inspection by HA as such is a routine activity to ensure quality although unannounced inspections are significant.

Certain other relevant permissions for a trial such as IP import, device import, biological sample import or export are granted by HA or other government bodies closely working with HA. These associated permissions should be applied along with the permission for trial conduct or once the trial approval has been obtained as per local regulations. HA inspection and approval may be a prerequisite for clinical sites to conduct a specific type of studies after meeting necessary requirements. For instance, Indian HA approval is a prerequisite for any clinical pharmacology unit to conduct trials in healthy subjects.

46.Documents for HA or EC permission

The clinical trial application consists of several documents along with the clinical trial protocol to enable the health authority or the ethics committee to review the proposal from a scientific and ethical perspective. Procedures and documentation requirements may vary among different authorities or ethics committees. Requirements may also depend on the nature of the compound, phase of drug development, indication, country of origin of the drug product and many other factors.

Here is a list of documents typically needed depending on the country, regulatory authority, and type of trial; however, this is not a comprehensive list. This is to give an overall impression of the nature of documents, which may be required.

Clinical study documents:

- Clinical study protocol
- Summary of protocol in national language
- Signed protocol signature page
- Informed consent form and translated copy in local language
- Investigator Brochure
- Justification for study entry criteria (inclusion/exclusion)
- List of study sites
- Data monitoring committee, data safety monitoring board, adjudication committee (composition, members, governing procedures)
- Declaration that the patient will have access to study drug after closure of the study
- Biological sample handling procedure (location, duration of storage, analysis to be performed and disposition plan)
- Serious adverse event data (patient identifiable data) archival procedure
- Investigator's notifications after the last investigator's brochure update
- Drug accountability log
- Drug administration manual

- Biological sample handling procedures
- Summary of available clinical data (if not part of Clinical Trial Application)
- Copies of references cited in the protocol
- Quality of life questionnaires, patient diaries, performance scales
- Patient reported outcome questionnaires in English, validated translations, certificates of validation
- Arrangement for subject recruitment (advertisements, radio scripts for subjects)
- Peer review of trial
- Ethical assessment made by the investigator
- Paper CRF copy or eCRF screenshots
- Trial data custodian details

Investigational medicinal product:

- Investigational medicinal product dossier (for European union and in some other countries): The IMPD includes summaries of information related to the quality, manufacture and control of the investigational medicinal product, data from non-clinical studies and from its clinical use. An overall risk-benefit assessment, critical analyses of the nonclinical and clinical data in relation to the potential risks and benefits of the proposed study have to be part of the IMPD.
- IND documents in the US: Introductory statement and general investigational plan, Investigator's brochure, protocols, chemistry, manufacturing and control information, pharmacology and toxicology information, previous human experience with the investigational drug. This is for opening an IND for initial investigation in humans for a new compound.
- GMP certificates and manufacturing authorizations for the manufacturers
- Certificate of analysis for the batch of products to be used
- Summary of product characteristics or approved drug label in case of commercial products used as comparator
- Importer's manufacturing authorization

- Certification of the QP (qualified Person) that the manufacturing plant works in accordance to GMP (applicable in Europe)
- Drug label (in local language)

Administrative documents:

- Form 1571 (in US)
- EudraCT Number (in EU)
- Country specific application forms and covering letters
- List of health authorities where trial application is submitted
- List of participating countries
- Key country approval letters or US ethics committee approval letter
- Copy of scientific advice
- Letter of authorization to act on behalf of the sponsor (in case regulatory activity is outsourced)

Vendor information:

- Central lab information (processing lab, point of contact in country, accreditations, lab director's CV and certificates)
- All external vendor information
- Transfer of obligations (in the US)
- Operational manual from vendors

Clinical Site /investigator/ethics committee:

- Facilities for the trial (facility write up)
- Trial facility approvals (if applicable)
- Audio-visual recording of informed consent (in India)
- Composition of ethics committee
- IRB registration, IRB SOPs (in India)
- Investigator's undertaking (India)
- Form 1572 (US)
- CV of the principal investigator, license to practice, certificates (for each site)
- CV of coordinating investigator, license to practice, certificates

- Information about sub-investigator, pharmacist and other study staff
- Local lab information (accreditation, lab director's CV, certificates)
- Indemnity or compensation in the event of injury or death attributable to the clinical trial
- Insurance or indemnity to cover the liability of the sponsor or the investigator
- Compensation to investigators
- Compensation to trial subjects
- Clinical trial contract between trial site, investigator and sponsor
- Insurance for trial subjects
- GCP training certificate of the investigators

47.Clinical trial application (CTA)

Clinical trial application (CTA) is a request to a health authority (HA) of a country seeking permission to conduct a clinical trial. Typically, it is in the form of a dossier with the trial protocol and other supportive documents along with a fee for review. CTA is the responsibility of the sponsor unless outsourced to a contract research organization (CRO). It is a coordinated effort to compile the dossier and could be complex depending on the structure of the regulatory department of the sponsor, country requirement or nature of submission (original submission or amendment).

All necessary documents are compiled in the prescribed format and quality checked prior to HA submission. The process begins with the identification of countries where the trial is planned. The next step is the identification of the documents required for each HA. Operationally, certain required documents could have dependencies; hence, planning is essential to meet timelines. For instance, IMPD, CMC or certificate of analysis documents are dependent on the availability of certain experiment reports, which in turn is dependent on the availability of drug product. In another example, informed consent form (ICF) and case report form (CRF) can be finalized only after the protocol is final.

Several functions are involved for the availability of different documents and their timelines should be considered in trial planning. Sometimes, certain documents are readily available while others need to be prepared specifically for a trial. Occasionally trials could be planned in a country due to minimal document requirement, especially in early phase development. In a well-managed setting, it may not be the bottleneck as the development program is planned in a comprehensive way considering all this.

Once the required documents are identified for the trial application, document availability is tracked. The process involves close follow up as several people, functions, and organizations may be involved. A quality check is included to ensure that the right documents and the correct versions are submitted to HA in the required format. HAs may also have a checklist to verify that the application is complete before accepting the application. Typically, organizations have internal SOPs to QC the dossier before submission.

The clinical trial application may be electronic and in such cases, the documents are submitted by uploading it to a web portal or submitting CD-ROM along with a cover letter. If the submission has to be made in the paper format, then required number of dossiers are prepared and submitted by courier or by hand as per the working practice of the authority. Typically, a fee is paid to the HA for review. An acknowledgement of the CTA submission is obtained for future reference and archival in the trial master file.

Other associated permissions for a trial such as import/export permits for biological samples and drug products may be processed by the HA or other government departments along with the clinical trial permission. The requirements for the trial should be evaluated and necessary permissions should be applied along with the CTA. At times, the regulatory affairs function may be outsourced to a CRO when the expertise is not available, or the sponsor doesn't have any representation in a country. A letter of authorization may be required for the CRO to work on behalf of the sponsor and liaise with the HA.

From a project management perspective, significant efficiency can be achieved through better planning, follow up and coordination to achieve the milestone of CTA submission. Approval timelines may be upto two months in many European countries, upto six months in many emerging economies including India or upto one year in China. In the US, a formal approval step is not required if an IND is open; otherwise, the trial can be initiated after a waiting period of 1 month. However, US FDA may come up with questions, request to hold the trial or request for amendment at any time. HA review timelines may also depend on the nature of the trial, the phase of drug development, risk/benefit proposition, unmet medical need, and so on. Understandably, it is easier to plan and conduct trials in countries with predictable regulatory timelines.

In multi-country trials and while dealing with health authorities with unpredictable timelines, early CTA filing is operationally desirable. At least one round of review and query/response cycle should be considered in timeline planning. Preparing responses to queries from HAs requires a co-ordinated effort involving different functions depending on the nature queries.

Depending on the nature of the trial, the lead time for approval, any uncertainly on approval and other factors, operational planning at the sites may progress. Trial setup can only proceed in full swing after securing HA permission.

48. Import and export license

In today's integrated world, clinical trial planning and conduct span beyond country and state boundaries. Many trial activities are carried out by organizations or units of multinational organizations situated in countries different to where the clinical sites are located. For instance, the drug product manufactured in the US may be imported to India for a clinical trial while the biological samples are shipped to China for bioanalysis. The data management and statistical analysis could be handled in another country. Many clinical trials (Phase II onwards) are conducted at multiple sites in multiple countries to meet recruitment or to utilize specific expertise.

In such scenarios, investigational products, biological samples, and other trial materials cross legal boundaries of different countries with differing provisions for handling these controlled substances. Permissions in the form of import/export license are required so that government officials allow passage of these shipments across legal boundaries. Whenever there is an export from a country X to country Y, an export license may be required from country X in addition to an import license from country Y.

The operational procedures and timelines for obtaining import or export license should be understood while planning a trial. The government authority, which deals with such permissions in a country, may be the drug regulatory authority or another authority dealing with foreign trade.

The trial materials to be imported or exported as well as the quantity should be evaluated during trial planning. Quantity calculation should consider possibilities of damage during shipment. For instance, a temperature sensitive drug shipment may be damaged due to temperature excursions in transit. The possible backup options in such eventualities should be explored for contingency planning in the light of the specific situation.

In certain critical circumstances, backup shipments may be kept ready for immediate shipment. Shipments in divided parts may be another option. In countries, where permissions can be obtained quickly, advance planning may not be necessary. Otherwise, permissions covering potential supplementary shipments should also be obtained.

The applications are typically made along with the clinical trial application; however, it could vary depending on the situation. For instance, ethics committee (EC) approval of the trial in the originating country may be a prerequisite for applying a permission to import biological samples to another country. Hence, an application could be made only after obtaining the EC approval. The import or export license may be valid for a specific duration and it needs to be reapplied periodically in long duration trials.

The data elements in the import and export license such as the name of the drug or quantity should be accurate and consistent with other study documents (e.g. protocol, certificate of analysis, etc.). It is prudent to get the applications or permissions reviewed by the regulatory affairs representatives or other relevant team members as errors may lead to problems in customs clearance.

When an amendment is made to the study protocol, the impact on the import/export license applications should be evaluated. For example, if there is a modification to the quantity or name of the drug to be imported, the license should be reapplied, or necessary amendments requested.

In a large multi-country and multi-center trial, the extent of import/export permit requirement could be very extensive with considerable resource and effort requirement. It also requires specific expertise and experience to understand country-specific regulations and standard work practice. Increasingly, such activities are managed through specialized service providers, who may also have capabilities to support the full range services and logistics of supply change management in clinical trials.

Electronic databases with information on requirements, timelines, and logistics are available for quick reference.

Examples of information, which may be required by the authorities:

License to import drugs:

- Importer details
- Name of drug and quantity
- Country of origin
- Study protocol number
- Rationale for quantity to import
- Undertaking to use the drugs as per good clinical practice (GCP)

License to export biological sample:

- Exporter details
- Type of application (type of trial)
- Name of drug used in the trial
- Purpose of sample export
- Type of sample
- Shipment details (port of loading, port of discharge)
- Address of laboratory where analysis will be performed

License to import biological samples from trials conducted in other countries:

- Ethics committee approval of the trial
- Informed consent form
- Export license from the originating country
- Undertaking in case export license is not required
- Material transfer agreement
- Name and address of the institution providing the samples
- Name and address of the institution where sample is sent
- Nature of biological material
- Number of samples and duration of shipment
- Purpose and need for sample transfer

- Type of research
- Category under which the infectious substance is classified
- Safety norms to be observed during transit and analysis
- Any risks with the transfer of samples
- Research standard (ICH, WHO, etc)
- Copy of memorandum of understanding between the parties
- Implications on any national health program
- Any implications for the scientific interest of the country

49. Medical monitor

As per ICH GCP, the sponsor has a responsibility to designate appropriately qualified medical personnel (called medical monitor) who would be readily available to advise on trial related medical questions or problems. If necessary, outside consultant(s) may be appointed for this purpose.

Many unforeseen circumstances may arise during a trial conduct that has to be addressed by the sponsor on a case by case basis. Sponsor's medical monitor guides the investigators on medical or scientific issues on behalf of the sponsor. Examples of typical issues, which come up for clarification or guidance, are:

- Clarification on scientific aspects of the protocol
- Clarification on trial interventions
- Subject eligibility
- Individual subject discontinuation
- Study stopping rules
- Concomitant medication
- Management of adverse events
- Decisions on protocol deviations
- Dose adjustment
- Review of SAEs arising in the trial and preparation of narrative in real time

The medical monitor is generally medically qualified and is required to have a thorough understanding of the protocol, trial interventions and disease condition under study to guide the investigators. He or she may be the medical expert involved in designing the trial or another staff member.

The medical monitor should forge a working relationship with the trial investigators and be available round the clock for emergencies. It is not uncommon to have a difference of opinion with the investigators and it should be managed professionally complying with good clinical practice principles with safety and interests of the subjects given primacy. The joint decision of the medical monitor and the investigator should be documented appropriately before implementation. Any steps for immediate subject safety should be allowed even if it is in deviation to the protocol.

Certain decisions can be implemented only through a protocol amendment. For instance, a subject failing entry criterion with borderline laboratory results should not be randomized even if it is medically reasonable. It may not be acceptable from a GCP perspective and hence, should only be implemented after a protocol amendment. The guidance of the medical monitor is not binding on the investigators. The ultimate responsibility for subject safety remains with the investigator.

The medical monitor also serves as a consultant for the trial team on the medical aspects of the trial. To facilitate interaction in a global setting, internet-based platforms are available where investigators and trial team can request clarification or ask questions to medical monitors. In such platforms, the responses as well as the entire question/guidance process is documented for future reference. It is particularly helpful for sponsors to review the questions from different investigators and the guidance provided in settings where the medical monitoring is outsourced. Such platforms allow workflow of the CRO's medical monitor escalating questions to sponsor's medical monitor when assistance is required.

Another key responsibility of the medical monitor is the review of subject data on an ongoing basis from a medical perspective. It ensures that the subject data looks plausible, and the trial management is as per protocol and standard medical practice. In this way, the medical monitor has a major role in data management and ensuring the safety of trial subjects. Any suspected deviations should be discussed with the trial operation team and the investigators as appropriate. A high-level oversight of the trial conduct with optimum quality is a typical expectation from medical monitors. Periodic review of key trial quality metrics along with the operations team is essential.

The role of medical monitors has evolved over the years as a key scientific interface between investigators and various stakeholders involved in trial conduct. The ability to balance between scientific expectations and operational realities while managing different stakeholders is often required. The sponsor's medical monitor could also serve as the spokesperson person for the sponsor on trial related questions.

50. Investigator

ICH GCP (good clinical practice) defines an investigator as 'a person responsible for the conduct of the clinical trial at a trial site. If a trial is conducted by a team of individuals at a trial site, the investigator is the responsible leader of the team and may be called the principal investigator.'

An investigator may be supported by one or more sub-investigators. As per ICH GCP, a sub-investigator is 'any individual member of the clinical trial team designated and supervised by the investigator at a trial site to perform critical trial-related procedures and/or to make important trial-related decisions (e.g., associates, residents, research fellows).'

In a large trial with multiple centers, there may be a coordinating investigator defined in ICH GCP as 'an investigator assigned the responsibility for the coordination of investigators at different centers participating in a multi-centric trial.'

Protecting safety and rights of the subjects participating in clinical trials is critical as per good clinical practice and the primary responsibility of an investigator to take all steps to safeguard it. The roles, responsibilities, and obligations of an investigator are clearly defined in ICH GCP and are out of the scope of this discussion.

Clinical trials in patient population are generally conducted by investigators who are practicing physicians. Often, the primary interest of the physicians is patient care or teaching, whereas clinical trial conduct is an additional engagement; it could be for monetary benefit or scientific interest. They may be working in an academic hospital or a general hospital. As most of the trials are conducted in referral hospitals, the investigators may have referring physicians who are primary physicians of the subjects. Additionally, investigators may recruit from their own patient pool.

Trials in healthy subjects are mostly conducted in clinical pharmacology units of contract research organizations (CRO), which are commercial organizations. Academic medical institutions may also have such facilities. Typically, the primary engagement of investigators in such centers is research work. Occasionally, practicing physicians work as investigators at these centers for additional engagement.

There are other specialized centers, where both clinical research and patient care get equal attention. It is important to understand the primary engagement and motivation of the investigators as this decides the attention, interest, and involvement required for successful trial conduct. Although investigators are typically medically qualified, there could be exceptions in some countries.

In such situations, other medically qualified investigators would be available to take any medical decisions.

Sub-investigators are typically residents, associates, junior doctors or consultants who assist the principal investigators in trial conduct. Sub-investigators handle much of the routine work, whereas, the principal investigators take the supervisory and decision-making responsibility. The delegation of responsibilities to sub-investigators must be appropriately documented in the delegation log. Sub-investigators have to be appropriately qualified and trained by the principal investigator and the sponsor commensurate with the delegated responsibilities. It is important to understand the professional relationship of the sub-investigators with the principal investigator and their primary engagement.

Coordinating investigators are generally key opinion leaders (KOL) in their therapeutic field and are from an academic background. They hold a say in the medical community, have physician following and have influencing capabilities. There may be country specific coordinating investigators or just one for the entire trial. Coordinating investigators play a major role in protocol development and investigator pool selection. It may be necessary to have such investigators in late phase or major therapy defining trials.

Type of institution, the source of funding, reputation, employment modality, and research culture in an institution determine the fundamental attitude of investigators towards research and thus, ease of conducting clinical trials at a given clinical site. Basic expectations of a sponsor from an investigator are practical feedback about the protocol, realistic estimate on recruitment, appropriate involvement in the trial process as well as compliance to GCP, ethical principles, and regulatory requirement. It is the sponsor's responsibility to select suitable investigators for a trial.

Investigator selection for a trial in healthy subjects with a known compound is generally simple. If new chemical entities (NCE) are to be evaluated in safety or tolerability trials (Phase I), investigator's technical skills, and experience should be carefully considered. The potential investigators need to have a thorough understanding of new drug development process and adequate professional experience of working with NCEs. The investigators should be able to characterize AEs properly and manage trial related emergencies.

Phase II or therapeutic exploratory trials in patients require a high level of involvement in protocol development and trial conduct. Clinical input from well-experienced investigators is invaluable for innovative adaptive trial designs. Typically, investigators who have adequate time and interest should be selected. As patients in these trials need to undergo a number of evaluations and frequent visits, attention from the investigators is crucial. Well-equipped research facilities are usually necessary for these trials.

Phase III or confirmatory clinical trials generally need a proportion of investigators with KOL status. These physicians get first-hand exposure to the investigational products in trials and may become active advocates of such therapies later. They play an important role in establishing the new medicines after approval. However, a majority of the investigators still need to be selected based on their capability to run a trial. Role of coordinating investigators may be indispensable, even though they may not contribute significantly to recruitment themselves. Generally, such trials can be conducted in many centers due to modest requirements. Such trials have high a likelihood of regulatory inspection; hence, experienced investigators/centers are preferred.

Phase IV or therapeutic use trials are close to routine medical practice, and may not require significant attention. Investigators with KOL status may be helpful if there is a sensitive objective such as comparison with a competitor's product. As these trials are often simple and straightforward, it may be a good platform for training and capacity building of new investigators. Typically, centers with basic facilities can handle such trials.

51.Site coordinator

Clinical sites have several supporting functions to assist the investigators in clinical trials. The site coordinator works as a project manager and as the name suggests coordinates among different functions and staff members at a site. He or she is also the point of contact for the sponsor and other external organizations working with the site on a trial. All communications to a clinical site are typically routed through the site coordinator and thus, serving as a bridge between the investigator and the sponsor.

Depending on the business model, the site coordinator may be appointed by the investigator or a site management organization. Well-structured contract research organizations (CRO) managing healthy volunteer trials generally have one or more project manager(s) to coordinate all trials from one sponsor. In a hospital practice setting, a sub-investigator, study nurse or pharmacist may work as a site coordinator along with other trial-related work.

The organization structure, primary responsibility and the mode of employment determine to a certain extent the professional approach of a site coordinator. A regular employee in a professionally managed organization whose primary job is project management would have a more professional approach and delivery standards than a student, who works part-time as a site coordinator in a trial at an academic hospital where sponsored research is of secondary interest. The expectation should be calibrated accordingly. Here is a set of activities, which the site coordinator may handle in different organizations depending on the business model and qualification of the person.

- Trial planning, setup and close out: Protocol development with sponsor, source document design, coordination for ethics committee submission, trial setup activities, point of contact for receiving trial supplies, coordination for site initiation, participation in investigator's meeting, resource planning for the trial, management of financial aspects of the trial, etc.

- Clinical research work: Trial subject identification, entry criteria assessment, informed consent form (ICF) discussion with subjects, schedule visits for subjects, clinical assessment, SAE reporting, etc.

- Coordination: Collaboration with sponsor, monitor, local and central laboratory, ethics committee, pharmacy, technical research staff members at the site, logistics group, data management group and service providers

- Monitoring activities and study progress: Investigator's file management, coordination for monitoring visits, participation in audits/inspections, and assessment of trial progress (e.g. enrolment, randomization, visit completion)

- Data management activities: Data entry into case report form (CRF) and query handling

The site coordinator should be skilful in communication, planning, problem-solving, and project management as well as proactive. Administrative skills add significant value to this role. He or she should be well accustomed to site's capabilities, local regulations, ICH GCP (good clinical practice), ethics committee requirements. Thorough understanding of the protocol and any specific trial requirements is important to guide the site team in day to day work.

It is common to be caught between expectations of the sponsor and performance of the site; thus, sound conflict management skill is essential. The study coordinator should be able to run the trial effectively with the available resources and manpower at the site. The coordinator should effectively collaborate with the study monitor to understand deviations or other issues in trial conduct and assist the site personnel to resolve it. Regular update to stakeholders on the trial progress is a key expectation.

52.Investigator management

Clinical trials in patient population are conducted at university hospitals, physician's clinics and private or public hospitals. Most sponsors prefer to have direct contact with investigators for running trials or consultation on study designs. Thus, it is important to forge and maintain a good working relationship with investigators for pragmatic planning, smooth trial conduct, faster recruitment and fewer quality issues. Certain specialized contract research organizations (CRO) have collaborations with hospitals to conduct trials in specific patient populations. Site management organizations (SMO) also mediate and facilitate trial conduct at clinical sites.

Organizations involved in clinical trials usually maintain databases with strategic information about investigators and clinical sites. Typically, there is a continued conscious effort in many organizations to identify, qualify and develop new investigators. Investigators are profiled based on qualification, facility, experience, attitude, time and interest. Periodically, investigators are categorized for suitability to a different type of trials.

A distinction may be made between a key opinion leader (KOL) and a key investigator (KI). While KOLs are influential, have physician following and have a say in the medical community, they may not be committed investigators. Thus, their contribution in terms of subject recruitment may be sub-optimal. Trial subject management is different from usual patient care and what is normal in routine practice may not be acceptable in the context a clinical trial. Sponsors often prefer to have KOLs in a trial for several reasons such as to bring credibility to the trial, provide first-hand experience to KOLs on new medicines, and get feedback on the trial design and so on. Many KOLs are also key investigators in a general sense.

In contrast, key investigators are major recruiters irrespective of their KOL status. The right mix of interest, time and commitment is crucial apart from access to patients and facility. In spite of growing acceptability of clinical trials in the society, only a small proportion of physicians are able to run sponsored trials satisfactorily. Some sponsors may have similar drugs in development and end up competing for the same set of investigators for similar trials. Thus, preferential access to investigators over competitors is desirable and continuous engagement is required to achieve that. A good working relationship, transparency, and trust between sponsor and investigator are essential for smooth trial conduct.

Here are a few common approaches to engage with investigators:

- Training new investigators who have interest and commitment to conduct trials
- Regularly conducting trials with same investigators
- Proactive consultation during trial planning
- Training of site staff on general aspects of clinical trials, audits/inspections, documentation, good clinical practice, etc. Sponsors typically have better a understanding of such topics and it may be of interest to the site staff.
- Helping the clinical sites in their own research or joint research in common areas of interest
- Joint publication of trial results
- Partner with investigators for capacity building at clinical sites to conduct innovative trials
- Create opportunities for investigators to discuss trial results in external forums
- Partner with investigators in community engagement programs on disease awareness

It is important to understand the motivation of investigators to conduct sponsored clinical research and tailor engagement approaches accordingly. Sponsors must be vigilant about conflicts of interest issues of investigators in the context of local regulations in their engagement with clinical sites. Typically, regulations have restrictions on the monetary and material benefit to investigators or institutions to prevent undue influence of commercial organizations.

It is not unusual to have circumstances of investigator dissatisfaction with the sponsors or partner organizations and its representatives. Such situations arise involving financial, cultural, procedural, communication and administrative factors. Often there is a clash of work culture i.e. a corporate way of working of the sponsor organizations vs. an academic way of working of investigators.

There is also a cultural clash in terms of patient care in routine practice vs. trial subject management with adherence to GCP and other regulations with extensive documentation. Newer investigators may be unfamiliar with the procedural or administrative framework of trial conduct. Investigators often don't realize the complexities of trial requirements until recruitment or find the various trial documents overwhelmingly extensive to follow.

Such issues should be anticipated and can be avoided to a considerable extent through proactive communication, training and repeated discussion of expectations. Background of the requirements and expectations should be clarified or brought into conversations as investigators may appreciate its importance when the rationale is provided. The value of periodic face to face interactions with a focus on professional relationship building is very important but is often underestimated.

Field monitors as the key interface with the clinical sites are at the forefront to manage the investigators. Medical monitors have an important role in managing investigators through the establishment of a medical and scientific connect.

53.Site management organization (SMO)

Site management organizations facilitate trial conduct at clinical sites in the setting of academic centers or hospitals. Such facilities have a primary focus on patient care or academic research. It may not be necessary to follow the rigor of GCP (good clinical practice) in academic research. Fundamentally, general patient management in routine medical practice could be broadly similar to subject management in a clinical trial barring strict requirement of protocol compliance or extensive documentation. Although many clinical sites are routinely involved in academic research, many of those don't meet the typical expectations of the sponsors.

Here are examples of expectation of sponsors from the clinical sites:

- Priority for clinical research activities
- Easy access to investigator and site staff
- Awareness of clinical trial processes, GCP, GLP (good laboratory practice), GDP (good documentation practice)
- Project management capabilities
- Precise estimation of recruitment capacity
- Special attention to trial subjects
- Availability of SOPs (standard operating procedures) for key processes
- Efficient logistics management capabilities
- Proper handling of trial supplies
- Availability of validated instruments
- Awareness of audits and inspections

Clinical research has evolved over time and many medical centers have adapted to integrate it into their routine work. Such centers have clinical research departments and study coordinators who take care of industry sponsored trials.

To help with centers that don't meet industry expectations, and hence remain unsuitable for sponsored trials, interfacing organizations have come up. Site management organizations (SMO) are contract research organizations (CRO) who work with clinical sites (hospitals, academic centers) to facilitate sponsored trial conduct and offer their services to sponsors. Operational model of SMOs widely vary. There are models in which SMOs set up the entire infrastructure at the investigator site for clinical trials along with trained manpower.

Generally, SMOs support administrative and logistic aspects of trial conduct at the sites. SMOs ensure appropriate site identification, GCP compliance, meeting recruitment targets, trial conduct within agreed budget, appropriate trial documentation, early identification of issues and overall supervision at the site. Scope of work varies as the trial progresses through different stages.

In the run up to trial initiation, the scope of work typically includes protocol and site feasibility assessment, site selection, contract negotiation, trial setup, logistics arrangement, informed consent form (ICF) customization, translation of essential documents, ethics committee (EC) dossier compilation, source data template preparation, assistance to investigator in pre-screening, training of site staff and preparation of the site for trial initiation.

During trial conduct, the activities are more of coordination with site staff, trial subjects, logistic service providers, sponsor, monitor, local and central laboratory, data management group, etc. The scope may include assistance in subject screening, consent process, subject follow up, documentation, investigator's file maintenance, subject reimbursement, adverse event reporting, protocol deviation reporting, EC notifications and data entry to case report form (CRF). Post study activities include data management work from site perspective, compilation and archival of investigator's folder, preparation of the site for closeout and coordination for audits or inspections.

SMOs typically appoint a study coordinator at the trial site to manage the trial. In some situations, the study coordinator may not be from the SMO and is directly employed by the investigator or the site. The SMOs may have certain SOPs or work practice documents to be followed at the trial site and could be helpful if the site does not have those processes. Those procedures should be reviewed along with the site staff and customized as necessary.

SMOs develop a good working relationship with many investigators in the course of managing trials for various sponsors. They can play a crucial role in site identification, feasibility evaluation and trial conduct. Some SMOs may have a network trial sites in several countries with or without therapeutic area specialization, which may come handy in swift trial setup in especially in large multicenter trials.

Here are few considerations while employing SMOs:

- SMOs should be employed sufficiently in advance during the protocol development
- Clarity on the scope of work as there may be overlap with the responsibilities of the sponsor and site personnel
- Any transfer of sponsor or investigator obligations or responsibilities should be appropriately documented
- Experience in the particular therapeutic area should be preferred
- Prior experience of the SMO with the investigator is an advantage
- Coordinators should be carefully chosen based on education, training and experience
- Complex projects should be handled by full time coordinators for a single study
- Study coordinators (if employed by SMOs) should be encouraged to forge working relationship with the site staff
- The SOPs of the SMO should be evaluated along with the site staff or investigator
- The training records of study coordinators should be reviewed
- Monitoring services should be selected from a different CRO to prevent conflicts of interest

- Any conflict of interest between the investigator, SMO and ethics committee should be considered

There are other organizations broadly providing similar services as an SMO but referred to as trial management organizations, investigative site networks, site alliance, etc. Generally, sites may align with SMO or similar organizations to have a better negotiating position especially in the absence of influential investigators. It is important to understand the dynamics of association of an SMO with an investigator.

54. Trial setup at clinical site

Trial setup is the preparatory work to make a clinical site ready to enrol subjects. Essential components are the execution of contract, ethics committee (EC) approval, training of site personnel as well as the availability of investigational products (IP), trial materials, case report form (CRF), active vendor services, randomization details, emergency code breaks and active insurance coverage for trial subjects. The important trigger to proceed with trial setup is approval from health authority (HA) and EC. Often, setup is initiated at risk in order to save time while the approvals are awaited. Operationally, it is a logistically intensive process.

Here are few factors, which may influence the approach:

- Number of clinical sites
- Number of countries
- Anticipated regulatory challenges
- Timeline challenges
- Budgetary constraints
- Material import/export requirements
- Mode of data management

- Complexity of evaluations in the trial
- Setup timelines of vendor services
- Infrastructure at the clinical sites

Trial setup must be completed before site initiation. It can be started after site selection or contract execution; however, the extent is largely dependent on the regulatory environment. Typically, EC and HA approvals are the key hurdles before study setup can proceed in full swing. For instance, IP cannot be supplied to a site unless all the approvals are in place.

Operationally, trials with single or few centers are easy to manage in terms of setup. Prioritization in consideration of available resources is crucial in multi-country or multicenter trials. It is usually not possible to initiate all the sites simultaneously due to regulatory and logistic limitations. Sites, which have better chances to recruit as per prior experience or any other assessment, are prioritized. The geographic location of the sites may also be a factor from logistics and cost perspective. Some centers or countries are considered backup options, and those are down on the priority list. Service providers must be informed about the prioritization plan for alignment.

Trials with complex protocols, which require multiple assessments, may be resource and training intensive. It may involve several service providers who would work with the sites for training, device installation or trial material supply. Service providers may have capacity limitations and thus, need to prioritize their work. Lead time of service providers for setup activities should be taken into consideration in project planning.

Project management tools are helpful to plan and track the progress at individual sites while managing multiple sites. Several milestones could be framed on the activities leading upto initiation such as document availability, translations, EC/CA submission and approval, budget negotiation, import/export permit application, contract execution and site training. It allows building metrics on progress at the trial or regional level for monitoring of progress. Some of these metrics could be part of contracts with service providers as milestones.

Budget negotiation and site contract may be by far the most cumbersome activity in the preparatory phase. Discussion with the sites on budget and recruitment targets should be undertaken early on when there is an option to choose other sites. Budget negotiation can be protracted as sites take time to understand the cost drivers, make specific grant requests and negotiate with the sponsors for a better fee structure. Considerable time may be spent in the back and forth discussions as well as in obtaining additional approvals within sponsor organizations. Any higher than provisioned budgets typically require review by financial, legal and compliance functions to prevent any breach of regulations.

Clinical trial agreements with the sites could be a lengthy process as it is reviewed and signed by the administrative head of the institution where the trial is planned besides the investigator. Overhead fees structure, schedule of payment, indemnification, insurance coverage of trial subjects, publication policy, intellectual properly, confidentially and privacy clauses, etc are the typical areas where there could be disagreement between organizations of sponsor and trial site. Legal and financial reviews are typically part of the process, and such functions in public institutions may have no stakes in the trials as such.

During trial conduct, it may become necessary to open new sites due to unsatisfactory recruitment at the existing sites. There are financial implications in adding each new site and initiating setup activity. When there is uncertainty on the approvals at a particular site, setup activities of expensive services may be deferred.

55.Biological sample collection accessory

Many evaluations in clinical trials require biological sample collection, especially in early drug development clinical research. The biological samples could be blood, plasma, serum, sputum, urine, stool, tissue biopsy, saliva, etc. Some of these samples need to be shipped to a central facility for analysis due to lack of expertise at the site, standardized evaluation at one laboratory or cost consideration. Appropriate trial materials or accessories are supplied to the sites for sample collection, processing, storage, and shipment.

The accessories could be empty sample tubes, labels, syringes, blood collection catheters, processing chemicals, laboratory manuals, help books, single page pamphlets with instruction on sample processing, storing, and so on. These are customized as per the trial requirements and/or complexity of the procedure. These trial materials are often supplied by the sponsor through a service provider (e.g. central laboratory). There may be a necessity of specialized instruments for sample collection or processing, and it may need to be supplied to the site.

The process of planning, securing permissions, and logistics is broadly similar to the process discussed in the section on IP supply. The sample handling procedures should be simplified, as the site staff may not have the expertise on laboratory methods. Collection tubes are typically color-coded or explicitly labelled for easy identification. Stepwise instructions should be prepared concisely for clarity at the sites. Single page quick reference flow charts are commonly prepared along with detailed manuals. It is a good practice to have all the details in a stepwise manner in the laboratory manual but minimizing such details in the protocol; only high-level information is required in the protocol. If outsourced, the central laboratory takes the responsibility of all this preparatory work and it should be initiated along with trial planning.

The clinical and laboratory personnel at the site should familiarize themselves with the accessories, laboratory manual, flowchart, and protocol. Typically, the central laboratory would work with the relevant site staff members for setup and training before site initiation. In case of complex procedures, demonstration and dry runs are helpful for familiarization and identification of any issues. Video instructions could be considered in a trial with a large number of sites. Compatibility of the accessories to the site instruments should be checked. For instance, the collection tubes may not fit into the centrifuge at the site. It is better to identify such issues early during feasibility or trial setup and address that in advance.

If the accessories need to be locally procured, it should be clarified explicitly with the clinical sites during feasibility evaluation. The site should begin the procurement process as soon as the draft or final protocol is available. When the clinical sites are involved in protocol discussion in the early stages, many of the issues could be identified and appropriately addressed. It is not unusual to discover minor but potentially disrupting issues at the time of trial initiation (e.g. non-availability of a vacutainer of particular volume or with a specific coagulant).

Meticulous labelling of the sample tubes is crucial to identification during shipment, storage or retrieval for analysis at various locations (site, laboratory) as well as data integrity after analysis. Pre-labelled tubes are often provided to the site; alternatively, labelling information may be provided in the protocol or sample handling manual and the labels are generated at the site. Quality control steps are necessary for this process. When certain processes are outsourced to other organizations (e.g. central laboratory), proper coordination is necessary. Import/export license requirements for these trial supplies should be evaluated and applied as necessary.

56.Study specific device setup at site

Devices may be used in clinical trials for drug administration, laboratory or physiologic assessments, remote monitoring of subject status and emergency safety measures. Trial medication may be administered by customized devices e.g. inhalers with a bronchodilator, insulin injecting devices. Syringe pumps are utilized for intravenous drug administration. Increasingly, telemonitoring technologies are utilized to collect data on blood pressure (BP), heart rate, mobility, physical and mental function, adverse events, quality of life and medication adherence directly from subjects at their homes, reducing or eliminating the need for visits to a study site.

Potential devices to be used in a trial are explored along with trial concept development. Literature, videos or live demonstrations may be requested from the service providers. The initial step helps to ensure that the devices would be able to meet the trial requirements. The general operational aspects to be clarified are cost, timelines, installation, qualification, calibration, site training, break down support, vendor operations in the target countries and data management. Import/export license requirements for between-country shipments should be evaluated. Setup timelines should be taken into account in overall trial planning.

The devices could be purchased or rented from service providers. Any required qualification of the devices at the site (installation, operation or performance) must be performed and documented. Device training of site staff should be completed before trial initiation as per contract with the service providers. In case of complex instruments, it is ideal to have an onsite demonstration, so that the site personnel are conversant with the device operation. The site personnel should also familiarize themselves with practice before trial initiation. Operational aspects are typically detailed in a separate manual in a stepwise manner with graphic illustrations. Videos on the device use are particularly helpful if available.

Operational aspects of device data handling should be discussed with the clinical site, service provider and data management team. Certain devices such as a drug administration pump, inhaler or external cardiac pacer may only have few or no data for reporting and it can be transmitted through case report form (CRF) if required. Devices such as an automated BP instrument or peak expiratory flow meter show the reading instantly in the inbuilt monitor. Such data can be noted in the source document and subsequently, reported through CRF.

In other situations, the device may record the assessment in an attached or inbuilt memory card (e.g. Holter recordings) and these data are transmitted to the service providers for central reading and interpretation. The transmission can be via the internet after downloading to a computer system or via telecommunication network in real time. It may be required to ship the memory cards for data download. The processed data is subsequently transmitted to the trial database directly with any involvement of the CRF in this process. The method and specifications of data transfer should be worked out before trial initiation. It is a good practice to have a test run of data transfer to identify programming errors prior to dealing with actual data.

In certain scenarios, after the central readout, the service provider is required to notify the investigator or the sponsor's medical monitor instances of clinical concern. The procedure should be worked out in terms of the format of alert, criteria for notification, recipients, and timeframe.

The data obtained from the devices may potentially unblind the trial due to suggestive pharmacological effects of trial treatments. Independent persons at the clinical site and in the data management team should be identified for such data handling. Dedicated computer terminals with password protection or other acceptable methods may be used to prevent access to such data.

Commonly used devices (e.g. BP instruments, thermometers, etc.) may be supplied to clinical sites for standardized measurement across the sites with centrally validated devices. Investigators may notice a difference in readings between the devices at their centers vs. the centrally supplied trial devices. It could due to several reasons such as a difference in the method of use, improper use or a problem with either device. It is a rather common issue, and it should be explored proactively for swift identification and resolution (if encountered). If such complaints are from multiple sites, there could be systematic issues. Any anticipated difference should be discussed with the investigators upfront for assurance.

57. Validation and calibration of instruments

Instruments used in clinical trials must be validated and calibrated to ensure suitability for intended use. The consistency of measurement accuracy is fundamental to the credibility of any experiment including clinical trials. Validation has been defined by Wikipedia as the process of establishing documentary evidence demonstrating that a procedure, process, or activity carried out in testing and then production maintains the desired level of compliance at all stages. Validation ensures that the instrument works to produce the intended result as per stated functional intent.

Validation includes qualification, which demonstrates that the instrument is properly installed, work correctly and lead to the expected result. The entire process of qualification involves design, installation, operational, performance and component steps.

Calibration has been defined by ICH as the demonstration that a particular instrument or device produces results within specified limits by comparison with those produced by a reference or traceable standard over an appropriate range of measurements.

While measuring key safety or efficacy endpoints in clinical trials, calibration of instruments is extremely important. This concept applies to all instruments used either at the laboratories or at clinical sites including those provided to clinical sites or trial subjects.

The method of validation and calibration as well as the frequency of calibration are determined by the manufacturer and are provided in the instruction manual or in another document. There are independent external organizations that are authorized to calibrate instruments and certify. However, it is not mandatory to have external organizations to perform calibration, and it can be handled internally following manufacturer's instruction.

Generally, laboratories can be expected to have such documentation, and it should be part of the evaluation process. Sometimes, such documentation may be requested by ethics committees. It is important to ensure the clinical sites are aware of such requirement.

Clinical sites should maintain schedule and certificates of calibration for all instruments in the facility. In relation to a particular trial, calibration records of the instruments to be used in the trial are of interest. It should be evaluated during site selection, initiation or any other routine monitoring visit. Typically, such documents are reviewed during an audit or inspection.

In situations where there are differences in the readings taken with centrally supplied but commonly used clinical instruments (e.g. thermometers, BP instruments, etc.) vs. locally used instruments, validation documents are helpful to assure investigators.

58.Central laboratory

Central laboratories (labs) may be engaged to manage certain aspects of one or more laboratory parameter assessments. Typically, it is a trial level and central arrangement for all clinical sites. The primary purpose is standardization by eliminating variations due to assessments at multiple laboratories. Other motivations could be expertise, resource, etc.

Various assessments could be managed through central labs such as safety, electrophysiology, imaging or biomarkers and so on. Biological sample handling and assessment commonly managed by central labs. Logistics is typically part of the services, but sometimes central labs are solely engaged to manage sample logistics. Conventionally, any lab that is arranged by the sponsor is called a central lab even though the trial has only one site.

The decision to engage a central lab should be taken carefully considering factors such as trial requirement, cost, expertise, geographic coverage, turnaround time, accreditation and capability to develop new methods if necessary. In general, central labs are expensive, and bring in additional administrative complexities to the trial management. Regardless of central lab use, there should be provision for local lab use for emergency safety evaluations. A central lab may have multiple analytical facilities at different geographic locations, and generally, this is not an issue if the processes have been standardized and are reproducible across the locations.

The requirement of central lab services is identified at the time of study protocol development. The scope, deliverables, and timelines are drafted into a standard work summary format for feasibility evaluation and competitive bidding. A draft protocol or concept sheet may be shared for a better understanding of requested service. When central labs have the specific expertise, a point by point discussion with the technical staff is essential and any suggestions should be considered in an open mind. It is imperative to ensure that the requirement is well understood, and any pertinent issues are clarified during the planning stage.

Several central labs may be involved in a trial and the scope may be limited or extensive. The services may be required from the time of screening or later in the trial. Proper planning and periodic review of setup ensure timely activation of services.

Central lab setup activities begin at the service provider's organization. A project manager is assigned to coordinate within and outside the organization. An operational plan is worked out in consultation with the sponsor taking both technical and operational elements in the form of a central laboratory specification. The following information is typically part of the specification document to describe the scope.

- Key relevant trial protocol elements
- Trial and central lab timelines
- Trial materials (accessories, devices, reagents, software)
- Development of any methods or processes and customization
- Preparation of customized test kits when necessary
- Training documents and lab manuals
- Logistics services
- Databases for lab data management
- Reconciliation plan with clinical database
- Helpline facilities
- Obtaining any permissions, licenses or approvals
- Supply of trial materials to site and device installations (if required)
- Site inventory management plan
- Site staff training requirement

The central lab specification may be an extensive document as the labs have templates to enable customization for a wide range of requirements from various sponsors. Typically, the central lab personnel prepare a draft for further review. A careful review of this document is essential to ensure study specific requirements are covered and unnecessary elements are not included.

The preparatory work takes time and it should be considered in trial planning. When multiple clinical sites are involved, prioritizing sites helps to optimize efforts. The central lab may sub-contract certain responsibilities to its partner organizations. For instance, sample shipment services would be further outsourced to courier agencies.

Training of site personnel should be initiated closer to trial initiation. The extent and mode of training depend on the complexity of the procedures and experience of the clinical site. Mode of training is decided on a case by case basis, and it could be through online materials, telephonic discussion or onsite training with a live demonstration. Training of field monitors on key aspects is equally essential for effective monitoring.

Logistics of central lab services are crucial for operational success. The arrangement should be process driven at each step such as shipment from a site, receipt at the lab, analysis, and reporting. Clinical sites should be provided with adequate information on how and when to contact the courier agencies as well as appropriate preparation for shipment. In some cases, subject visits might have to be planned to accommodate sample shipment schedule or vice versa when samples need to be shipped immediately.

The central lab must arrange for swift receipt of samples and subsequent handling. Despite volumes of samples from several sites, identification of every sample of each subject has to be maintained. Barcode incorporated labels are often utilized for tracking the sample movement. Some samples need to be analyzed and reported in an expedited manner for real-time decision making (e.g. entry criteria verification or adverse event determination). For certain evaluations (e.g. electrophysiology recordings), physical shipments may not be involved, and the recordings can be transmitted over the internet by uploading the data to specific web portals.

Data management is a key preparatory activity in this context. Individual reports may be necessary at the clinical site for real-time decision making. Notifications are commonly required by the sponsor for safety monitoring. Generally, reports are sent to the investigator or sponsor through emails, fax or courier. The labs may also set up online portals where the reports can be accessed remotely on a real-time basis. In blinded trials, reports must be appropriately customized to maintain blinding. Generally, central lab data is directly imported to the sponsor's analysis database as per data transfer specification.

With the high penetration of internet services, sample movement tracking electronically has become the norm to have better control, real-time tracking and minimize errors due to manual work. For instance, central lab database is set up to expect a certain number of specific samples (aliquots) for individual subjects at specific visits. The sites complete an electronic requisition form with specific details and use barcode labelled tubes. The central lab also uses barcode readers to receive these sample tubes and direct it for storage or specific analysis as predefined. It is usual to have different types of samples, analyses and storage requirements for different visits or subsets of subjects in a trial. The sample movement can be tracked real times in web-based platforms, and it is reconciled with sample collection data in clinical database or results in the analytical database.

The central lab manual and simplified flowcharts are usually developed to provide the necessary information or instruction to the clinical sites. These documents should be simple with clear, concise and pictorial illustrations in a stepwise manner. Video instructions may be also considered in certain situations.

It is not uncommon for site staff to make errors as they follow normal practice instead of trial specific requirements while handling samples (e.g. plasma separation when whole blood has to be shipped to the central lab). Similarly, it is important to ensure that samples are appropriately handled or stored at the central labs. Inadvertent errors may occur especially while dealing with large volume of samples or in long duration trials.

Such issues should be anticipated and monitored early on in the trial.

59.Investigational drug supply and storage

The ICH GCP (good clinical practice) has stipulated principles on supply and handling of investigational drug products (IP). Essential responsibilities of the sponsor are (i) IP supply to the investigators only after all the approvals are in place (ii) timely supply of the IP (iii) Ensuring the institutions to follow written procedure for handling and storage of IP (iv) Documentation of shipment, receipt, disposition, return, and destruction of IP (v) Maintenance a system for retrieving the IP or disposition of unused medication (vi) Ensuring the stability of the IP over the period of use and (vii) Maintenance of sufficient amount of IP to reconfirm specifications where applicable. Points (v) and (vii) have been described separately in other sections of this book.

IP supply is planned along with conceptualization of the trial, identification of target countries and sites. The trigger for IP packaging and shipment may vary among organizations depending on the flexibility, trial design, maturity of drug development program, the scale of trial and country-specific regulations where the trial is planned. As per ICH GCP, IP can be supplied to investigators only after all the approvals are in place (competent authority, ethics committee, and any other applicable approvals). This approach safeguards against any potential misuse of IP. Special trade zones may exist in countries which can be used to ship IP in quarantine condition even before the availability of the approvals. Subsequent release and use can be initiated only after obtaining all the approvals.

If IP has to be imported from another country, import permissions may be required, and this is typically linked to the competent authority approval of the trial. Even within a country, permission may be required for crossing legal boundaries of different states. Considering the sensitivity, organizations typically have an IP supply authorization step prior to any IP shipment to trial sites. Thus, IP supply is triggered after thorough verification of the approvals and legal requirements by authorized personnel (typically from regulatory affairs group). As per ICH GCP, it is the responsibility of the sponsor to promptly supply IP to the clinical sites. Hence, the sites are initiated after IP availability at the clinical site or in a nearby warehouse.

IP supply is a logistically intensive process and could be challenging for between-country shipments. The sponsor may handle this entirely or outsource part of it to service providers. IP can be supplied directly to the clinical sites; alternatively, it may be sent to a country level warehouse for storage, release or trial-specific repackaging and labelling before shipment to the sites as necessary. Several people from various organizations are involved in this multi-step process. In a typical international shipment, the shipper collects the IP along with necessary documents (export permit, invoice, etc.) and confirms with their counterparts in the receiving country for the availability of required permissions (import permit). Once the shipment has been made, the air waybill, timing of shipment as well as expected time of arrival are notified to the receiving party. The shipment is custom cleared and shipped to the consignee.

Special attention is required for environment-controlled shipments. Specially designed containers are used along with continuous temperature and humidity recording during transportation. Storage conditions are specified on the containers and the invoices for ready reference. Typically, airport terminals have facilities to keep the shipments at proper conditions until further transport. If needed, gel pack or dry ice is replenished by the shipping agency before transfer to the consignee. The central pharmacy or clinical site must be intimated in advance to receive and store the IP appropriately. Holidays and weekends should be taken into consideration. Typically, shipments within a country are easier.

At the clinical site, the IP is thoroughly inspected for identification, condition after shipment as well as accountability against the invoice and other documents. Temperature and humidity data from data loggers is reviewed to verify proper transit conditions. Any discrepancy in quantity, damage of IP or temperature excursions should be documented and brought to the notice of the sponsor's authorized representatives. Typically, limited fluctuations may be acceptable based on the stability data; however, that specific guidance can only be provided by the sponsor or the manufacturer. Finally, the IP should be stored appropriately as per the invoice, drug label or manufacturer's instruction. Temperature and humidity monitoring are usually necessary until disposal.

Documentation related to transit (air waybill, invoice, receipt as well as verification at the site or central pharmacy, temperature and humidity recordings) is archived in the trial master file as evidence of transport in proper conditions. Similarly, storage condition data is required to confirm IP was appropriately stored until dispensing or destruction. Temperature and humidity data can be available graphically or as listings depending on the recording device configuration. Typically, all these data are also reviewed by the field monitor at periodic intervals and reported in the monitoring report.

Sometimes, medication available in the market may be used as comparative treatment, rescue medication or interacting drug in drug-drug interaction trials. It may have to be procured by the investigator locally as per the arrangement. Invoice of purchase and other documentation as applicable (e.g. certificate of analysis from the manufacturer) must be archived. Such medications should be transported and stored as per the label of the manufacturer.

In certain trials, IP is resupplied at periodic intervals (trials with multiple sites, long duration or competitive recruitment, IP with short shelf life). The clinical sites should be trained in the process of resupply and the lead time after a request. The inventory at the clinical sites should be periodically reviewed for any resupply requirement. Electronic inventory management systems may be utilized for ready access to the inventory. Such systems integrated with Interactive Response Technology (IRT) plays a vital role especially in large multisite trials in simplifying and automating many of these steps along with necessary documentation of IP accountability electronically.

60. Investigational product label

Investigational products (IP) used in clinical trials must be properly labelled according to local regulations. The requirements may vary from country to country and strict compliance is a legal obligation. In this section, drug label refers to the printed information on the primary, secondary, or tertiary packaging that helps in correct identification of IP.

Primary packaging is the immediate cover and the holding material of unit drug product. For tablets, it could be the blister or the bottle, which holds individual tablets. Secondary packaging holds a set of individual units e.g. a pack having 5 sets of 10 tablet blisters. Tertiary packaging is usually used for bulk medication transport and storage. It holds several secondary packages of drugs.

IP during transit through country borders is scrutinized by government officials of different countries and regions. Finally, it is dispensed to trial subjects and accountability of each unit is kept. Although, IP labelling is intended for identification, scenarios may be a bit different in blinded and controlled trials.

Purpose of IP labelling ensures the safety of subjects through correct identification, traceability, and facilitation of intended use. Name of sponsor, dosage form, route of administration, batch number, storage conditions, period of use (manufactured date and expiry date), directions for use, trial subject number, name of investigator, trial reference code, name of trial site and any applicable statutory warnings (e.g. keep out of reach of children, for clinical trial use only) are usually the labelling elements. It may vary depending on the country, trial design, IP, and local regulations.

Labelling requirements equally apply to marketed medicines or placebo used as comparators in a clinical trial. In certain situations, IP is supplied in bulk to the clinical site where subject specific packs are prepared. Labels are prepared at the site in such cases. Sample labels may require approval by the ethics committee and competent authority before use. Marketed medications procured from another country may need to be relabelled as per the requirement of the country where the trial is planned.

It is not unusual to have different names for one compound e.g. chemical name, generic name, and company given code name. Marketed products may have a brand name in addition. It is important to have a consistent naming convention of the IP in label, protocol and other related documents such as import/export permit.

Often, IP is prepared in one country to be used in another country where labelling requirement may be different. Labelling standards typically follow the local requirements (where IP would be used), irrespective of the country of manufacture. It should be considered especially while preparing individual patient packs. IP label for patient-specific packages may be needed in local languages. In a multi-country trial, the label can be prepared in a booklet format that has labels for different countries. Drug label preparation activity is led by drug supply functions and is typically reviewed and approved by a cross-functional team that includes regulatory functions with local knowledge.

Special planning is required in blinded trials to maintain traceability despite blinding. In bioavailability or bioequivalence trials, where different formulations of one compound are compared and traceability is crucial, identical duplicate tear off labels may be pasted on the subject files after drug administration; the original label remains on the empty unit dose package. Barcodes are also commonly used in labels to support accountability accurately. For example, when a subject receives a treatment in the trial site, the barcodes in the subject ID and the drug label could be scanned to record treatment administration.

61.Subject and Investigator compensation

Subjects taking part in clinical trials need to spare time, put in efforts and may incur monetary expenses to meet trial obligations. Healthy subjects gain no direct benefits, patients may potentially get direct benefits in terms of access to newer therapies and free healthcare (although temporarily). In placebo-controlled trials, patients allocated to placebo arms don't get any treatment-related direct benefit while they may be inconvenienced to some extent due to withholding of effective treatments. Expenses may be incurred due to loss of wage, travelling cost, phone bills, and so on. Subjects may also have to tolerate inconveniences while following trial restrictions.

Subjects are compensated monetarily towards their trial obligations; hence, ethical concerns arise as it may unduly influence them to take part in trials. As per good clinical practice

(GCP), compensation should be only towards reasonable expenses of participation and not as an enticement. Investigators are also paid for their time and the resources of the institution used in the trial. The fundamental difference between subject and investigator compensation is that investigators are paid for their professional service. There have been similar concerns about investigator compensation as discussed earlier for subject compensation.

Components of trial subject compensation are (i) loss of wage due to the trial (ii) travel costs (iii) any other specific expenses for the trial. Components (ii) and (iii) may be reimbursed on an actual basis after verification of invoices. Components of investigators' compensation are (i) investigator's fees (ii) trial setup cost (iii) subject hospitalization cost (iv) expenses for any equipment or device (v) expenses of screen failures (vi) treatment cost for adverse events (vii) ethics committee review costs (viii) expenses for shipment of samples or trial materials (ix) establishment fees or overhead expenses (x) compensation paid to trial subjects (xi) expenses towards salary of site staff (xii) purchase of consumable items. The components cited here are only examples and is not a comprehensive list.

Trial site costs under various headings can be broadly divided into two categories (i) milestone payments and (ii) trial related expenses paid to third parties. Depending on the business model, institutional policy and local practice, milestones may be different. Often, millstones are set in terms of subjects reaching specific stages in the trial such as screening, randomization, specific visits, or study completion. Database lock is often a milestone for investigator fees. It is not unusual to have a few complex calculations considering all costs for preparing an invoice. The second category of expenses is the cost incurred due to the purchase of goods or services for the trial from third parties such as cost of buying study specific instruments, shipment charges or treatment costs of adverse events. At the beginning of the trial, it is a common practice to pay in advance a setup fee, which is later adjusted based on actual expenditure.

While high compensation has the potential to entice subjects to trials for monetary benefits, low compensation may be discouraging for voluntary participation. It may be disproportionate to the loss of wage, trial-related expenses or the time and efforts needed for a trial. Subject compensation is a sensitive topic and should be carefully decided taking local factors into consideration. Ethics committees (EC) review and approve the compensation planned for subjects to ensure a balance. In general, investigator's fees are not reviewed or approved by the ECs or competent authorities.

In certain countries, investigators fees are requested by competent authorities or ECs for review to ensure the trial is well funded to meet its obligations. Typical concerns from ECs are around compensation for trial related injury, treatment costs for trial-related adverse events, investigator indemnity, etc.

Subject compensation is typically prorated and is linked to completion of specific visits. It ensures that subjects don't take undue advantage of the full compensation for limited participation. In some places, if subjects are withdrawn by the investigator due to any medical reasons, a full payment is made and if subjects drop out due to personal reasons, the payment is prorated. Other reasonable trial related expenses such as travel costs are compensated on an actual basis; however, there may be pre-specified upper limit. The mode and prorated schedule are specified in the informed consent form (ICF) and is explicitly clarified to the subjects before enrolment. Any cost to be incurred by the subjects during participation in a trial must be stipulated in the ICF and discussed with the subjects.

Although a loss of wage is one of the bases of subject compensation, wages of individual subjects are not taken into consideration, as it is tedious and impractical. In general, an average or minimum wage in the locality may be taken into consideration. Country-specific guidance may exist for compensation calculation. ECs may also have such guidance in the locality or in the concerned institution. In certain countries, compensation is not allowed for trial subjects who are patients.

Similarly, there may be restrictions on the total amount a subject can earn in a year through trial participation. Such restrictions should be considered and discussed with the sites. The clinical site should keep proper documentation of payments made to subjects and archive invoices if payment has been made against it.

Sometimes, compensation is the limiting factor in recruitment as subjects find it inadequate. It is particularly true in case of trials in healthy subjects who don't get any direct benefit otherwise. In such situations, the compensation may be revised after due considerations. However, it can only be implemented after EC approval. Investigator fees may vary among different clinical sites and countries. Typically, it is negotiated separately with each investigator. Compensation to the investigators should be kept confidential as per the contract. It may be necessary (depending on local regulations) to state in the ICF that the investigator is financially compensated for the trial; the exact investigator's fees need not be specified.

Analytics services are available to help with estimation of the subject and investigator compensation in different regions or countries taking into consideration previously negotiated similar studies. Once a draft protocol or synopsis is available, the basic parameters of the study in terms of target countries, trial population, visit structures, procedures, duration, etc can be the basis to get the first estimate. This forms the basis for further negotiation with the sites.

A detailed breakdown of the compensation should be provided to the investigators. It is a good practice to ensure that the investigators have understood the various components of the budget proposal in the context of trial protocol requirements and obligations. This is particularly important for long-term trials where investigators need to manage the budget over a long period.

62.Public domain registration of clinical trial

In an effort to bring transparency, basic information on clinical trials is required to be made accessible to the public. Typically, sponsors or investigators publish trial information in government-run websites, which are freely accessible over the internet. One of the goals is to have results of all trials available to other physicians or investigators and patients. In general, trials with negative result are not readily published in medical journals. Thus, an alternate platform was felt necessary.

There are international or country-specific websites to publish trial information. ClinicalTrials.gov (US), ctri.in (India), anzctr.org.au (Australia and New Zealand), and eudract.ema.europa.eu (European Union) are some of the websites where the trials are posted. Details of procedure, time of publication, applicability to individual trials, data elements to be published and periodic update requirements vary among different websites.

For ClinicalTrials.gov, applicable clinical trials, in general, include interventional trials (with one or more arms) of drugs, biological products, or devices those are subject to US FDA regulation, which means that the trial has one or more sites in the US, involves a drug, biologic or device that is manufactured in the US (or its territories), or is conducted under an investigational new drug application (IND) or investigational device exemption (IDE). Typically, trials in patients are published while trials in healthy subjects may not require publication. In other websites listed above, all trials are posted irrespective of the subject population. However, the requirements could change over time and need to be reviewed while planning a trial.

Publication of trial information can be a regulatory requirement and it may be necessary before enrolment in the trial. The responsibility mostly lies with the sponsor. In some instances, the investigator may be responsible, especially when he or she is also the sponsor. Elements of the disclosure are typically about the sponsor, investigational product (IP), trial protocol, concerned regulatory authority or ethics committee, study results, contact details of the sponsor, etc.

For example, the high-level data elements for ClinicalTrials.gov include title of the trial, background, interventions, ethics committee review and approval, data monitoring committees, oversight authorities, sponsor (name, organization, contact information), study description, status (record verification date, overall recruitment status, etc), study design, groups and interventions, conditions, keywords (for search), entry criteria and clinical site contact details. The trial progress is periodically updated including the results once available.

The trial disclosure in public domain may have implications on intellectual property. Typically, sponsors are cautious about revealing sensitive information to competitors. An intellectual property attorney or lawyer and other relevant personnel should review the data before posting. In addition, Accuracy of data must be verified. Operationally, those review processes and timelines should be taken into consideration.

Many organizations have specialized functions (e.g. disclosure office) to lead this activity. Once the publication requirements have been decided, a final protocol or a study report depending on the stage of the trial is the basis to draft the publication text. This is reviewed by subject matter experts, regulatory colleagues, and intellectual property attorneys to ensure technical accuracy, regulatory compliance, and non-disclosure of avoidable sensitive information. The trial project managers are responsible to update the progress of the trial through disclosure office. Third party service providers are also available to support this activity in an outsourced setting.

63.Investigator meeting

Traditionally investigator meeting (IM) are planned in large multi-centric trials. The primary aim is to discuss scientific and operational aspects of the trial in an interactive manner with the investigators and key clinical site staff. Clinical trials are complex undertakings and site staff needs to be familiar with the considerable amount of information specific to each trial. Reputed clinical sites are typically involved with multiple trials from various sponsors. IMs are opportunities where the investigators and site staff spend the time to focus on a specific trial and clarify any questions about the trial.

IM is different from site initiation visit (SIV) meeting, which has been discussed separately. The time of the meeting is typically prior to SIV if individual sites. Multiple IMs may be planned in long duration trials before and during the trial conduct. Such meetings are also helpful for protocol development in complex phase 3 trials.

A location is chosen carefully to minimize travel time, cost, and potential distraction. Separate IMs could be organized for investigators at different geographic locations. Preparation may take few months depending on the number of investigators and their geographic locations. Involvement of external event management organizations is common; large companies typically have specialized functions to coordinate the planning.

Participants, topics, and format need to be carefully chosen and are often key factors to the success of the meeting. It is important to keep in mind that experienced sites often attend IMs in the context of other trials and sponsors, and similar operational topics are discussed there. While planning the IMs, key goals to be achieved and incorporation of adult learning method should be considered.

Typically, the meeting duration is one to two days. The principal investigator, a sub-investigator, and a study co-ordinator from each clinical site as well as key members of the clinical trial team of the sponsor and the CROs participate in IM. A mix of scientific and operational topics are discussed such as the clinical development plan, protocol, safety of IP, SAE reporting procedure, timelines, enrolment strategy, GCP, randomization, blinding, IP handling, monitoring, data management, publication policy, communication between sponsor and site staff, etc. A separate training session for the trial monitors is often part of the IM.

Simple agenda, minimization of redundant topics, shorter presentations with interactive sessions, the scope for Q&A, focus on the protocol and key operational topics, use of audience response systems and audio translation facility to local languages are viewed positively. A common session with all participants and breakout sessions for a focussed group of participants are typically organized. IMs are typically video recorded for the benefit of non-participating site personnel. A short questionnaire survey may be conducted weeks in advance to find major areas of lack of understanding of the investigator, site personnel or other key trial team.

A considerable amount of time and effort is spent on IMs from both the sponsor and clinical site perspective. There is concern about the productivity of IMs given the significant amount of time, effort, and money spent on such events as pharma R&D budgets are under constant scrutiny. In general, IMs are viewed positively by the site staff and sponsors.

Investigators find IMs useful with opportunities for scientific networking and learning from more experienced investigators. Questions raised by certain sites may be helpful for others. This is also an opportunity for face-to-face interaction and engagement to foster a sense of team among different stakeholders. Occasionally, investigators bring up unnecessary topics such as the budget for discussion inappropriately; the sponsors' representatives should be prepared to manage such situations.

187

Web-based IM in virtual space have been tried in recent years to minimize cost, however, this is not yet popular enough to replace the conventional format fully. Technical glitches in connectivity and inferior quality of interactions have been typical issues. A mixed format with certain repetitive topics (e.g. GCP) in a web-based format and key unique topics (e.g. protocol) in face-to-face meetings could be an alternate approach. Web-based formats should be concise, simple, and interactive.

64.Site initiation

Site initiation is a formal step, in which the sponsor authorizes a clinical site to begin enrolment in a trial. It is planned after a careful evaluation of study setup activities in consultation with the site staff, monitor, and other vendors. Broadly, it consists of a review of study procedures and preparedness for trial conduct. Sponsors may complete a checklist at this stage to ensure compliance with regulations. Here are the typical prerequisites for site initiation.

- Health authority and ethics committee approvals
- Import and export licenses
- Contract with the clinical site and vendors
- Site selection report
- Verification of qualification of investigators and laboratory directors
- Financial disclosures of investigators
- Insurance for trial subjects
- Publication of trial information in public domain as applicable
- Active services of outsourced work (e.g. central labs, IVRS, courier services)
- Investigational products (IP) at the site
- Availability of case report form (CRF) for data entry

- Active monitoring services
- Training of study staff
- Readiness of the site in terms of manpower, infrastructure and any local arrangements to support the trial conduct

Once a proposed date of the meeting is available, an initiation agenda is prepared by the sponsor and shared with the site, monitor, and other relevant service providers. All trial personnel at the site (investigator, sub-investigators, pharmacists, study coordinator, laboratory personnel) should attend and participate actively in the initiation meeting. Sponsor's trial team should attend the meeting in person or through telephonic or video conference as considered appropriate. The monitor generally participates in person. Representatives of service providers may attend the meeting if required. A meeting attendance log is completed for the trial master file (TMF) filing purpose.

The agenda typically includes discussion on the study timelines, protocol, IP, informed consent process, CRF completion process, monitoring procedure, source data verification process, IP handling requirement, adverse event management and reporting, sample handling procedure, randomization procedure, emergency code break procedure in a blinded trial, potential sponsor and regulatory audits, good clinical practice (GCP), study documentation management, record keeping and publication of trial results.

Most organizations would have standard procedures to conduct an initiation meeting. Any outstanding issues should be discussed, clarified, and documented. Site preparedness to conduct the trial is reviewed with the monitor, investigator, and other site personnel. The investigator's file (IF) is reviewed for the availability of all documents required prior to trial conduct.

After the initiation meeting, the sponsor's study manager should review the situation with the monitor and the investigator/coordinator and take a decision on the authorization of enrolment. The initiation meeting minutes and the decision on trial authorization is formally communicated to the investigator in a written document. If significant deficiencies are observed, enrolment should be postponed pending corrective measures. The identified issues should be followed up and the situation reviewed later. Any training needs or pending setup activities should be addressed in the meantime by the responsible parties.

The monitor prepares a report on each site initiation visit documenting activities of the day, site preparedness along with narration of outstanding issues and the resolution plan. The report typically includes a checklist illustrating an overview of the situation. Outstanding issues are followed up in the next monitoring visits for resolution and documented in the corresponding visit report appropriately.

Often, at the time of initiation meeting, the investigators and site staff get to know the details of the trial procedures and requirements. As they start to imagine the operational aspects, several practical questions can be anticipated including a request for protocol modifications. At this stage, although the protocol is reviewed to refresh the understanding, no protocol modification is easily possible. Any change at this stage would need fresh cycles of review and approval. This must be explained at the outset. Nonetheless, every effort must be made to clarify any aspect of the protocol or study procedure as necessary.

Many of these activities could be managed by the CRO in an outsourced setting with minimal involvement of the sponsor's personnel. However, at this time it is prudent for the sponsor's project manager to closely review the progress with the CROs because critical issues may be found as the sites start to prepare for trial conduct. Any pertinent issues raised in one SIV may be important to be discussed during SIV at other sites in a multi-center trial.

65.Good documentation practice (GDP)

Documentation is a cornerstone of good clinical practice (GCP) in clinical trials. As a ground rule, it is believed, not anything that has not been documented has ever happened. Due to the history of fraud in clinical research and its potential implications on trial integrity, authorities are sensitive to good documentation practices. Once a trial is over, adequate documentation helps to reconstruct the events sequentially to reconstruct the trial conduct. It is crucial from a trial operation perspective, and it should be considered at each stage of the trial by all involved.

Here are a few relevant terminologies in this context from ICH GCP guideline:

- Documentation: All records, in any form (including, but not limited to, written, electronic, magnetic, and optical records, and scans, X-rays, and electrocardiograms) that describe or record the methods, conduct, and/or results of a trial, the factors affecting a trial, and the actions taken.
- Essential documents: Documents which individually and collectively permit evaluation of the conduct of a study and the quality of the data produced
- Source data: All information in original records and certified copies of original records of clinical findings, observations, or other activities in a clinical trial necessary for the reconstruction and evaluation of the trial. Source data are contained in source documents (original records or certified copies).
- Source documents: Original documents, data, and records (e.g., hospital records, clinical and office charts, laboratory notes, memoranda, subjects' diaries or evaluation checklists, pharmacy dispensing records, recorded data from automated instruments, copies or transcriptions certified after verification as being accurate copies, microfiches, photographic negatives, microfilm or magnetic media, X-rays, subject files, and records kept at the pharmacy, at the

laboratories and at medico-technical departments involved in the clinical trial).

ICH GCP guidance has listed the documents that should be available and archived by the sponsor and the investigator before, during and after trial conduct. Documents are filed in the trial master file (TMF) at the sponsor's office and at the investigator's file (study file), subject file or other locations at the clinical site depending on the working practice. The study manager or a designated associate at the sponsor's office and the investigator, study coordinator or a designated person at the clinical site are responsible for maintaining it. The document transfer between the sponsor and the investigator may occur via the monitor or directly depending on the arrangement. There should be agreement on the archival location of original documents. Both the sponsor and the site may have copies of these documents as per ICH GCP or local guidance as applicable.

The type of source document (hard copy or electronic) at the site, methods, and facilities for documentation and archival are explored during site feasibility evaluation. An agreement is signed at the time of site initiation (or before) for the locations of various trial documents at the site. Not all the documents may be available in the investigator's file (study file) or subject file for practical considerations depending on the working practice. For instance, drug accountability documents may be only available in the pharmacy. However, it may be a good practice to have general study-related documents in the investigator's file and individual subject related documents in the subject file.

Hospitals may have a record-keeping policy that is not in line with requirements of clinical trials, especially for patient records. In such cases, photocopies of the patient records (attested by the investigator) may be specifically archived in the subject file. Such issues should be discussed and clarified during feasibility or before trial initiation. If the site uses electronic source document systems, it should be verified for completeness, accuracy, reliability, validation, controlled access, audit trail in case of data modification, appropriate standard operating procedures (SOP) on its use and availability of data backup procedures. Sponsors should evaluate electronic systems at the investigator's site for appropriateness before authorizing its use.

The information required to be documented about the subjects' medical conditions, their illness history, treatment, protocol adherence, progress, or adverse events is typically exhaustive in comparison to routine clinical practice. Thus, it is important to understand the data requirements for the case report form (CRF) before trial initiation. In procedure intensive trials, it may be worthwhile to create study-specific source data templates keeping in mind the CRF, in addition to routine requirements. For instance, it may not be required to document the absence of certain illnesses explicitly in routine practice, whereas this is required in the setting of a clinical trial. It is generally required to explicitly document reminders, phone calls or adherence to restrictions in the subject file. Development of study specific source data template is particularly important in healthy subject trials.

Subject's illness history is an important component of entry criteria. Trials are typically conducted in referral centers and thereby, not all previous health records may be available. Subjects might produce copies of health records from their primary physicians or it may be requested by the investigator. Careful history taking and documentation is an important step, especially in cases where medical records are not available. Such issues should be discussed with the investigator or staff before trial initiation.

As per ICH GCP guidance, the investigator should maintain adequate and accurate source documents and trial records that include all pertinent observations on each of the site's trial subjects. Source data should be attributable, legible, contemporaneous, original, accurate, and complete. Changes to source data should be traceable, should not obscure the original entry and should be explained if necessary (e.g., via an audit trail).

It is good practice for clinical sites to have SOPs on good documentation in the source documents. In paper documents, the writing should follow ALCOA principle for data integrity i.e. attributable (clarity on the writer's identity through initials and signatures), legible, contemporaneous (i.e. the documentation time should fit the timeframe of the trial events taking into consideration acceptable or justifiable delays), original and accurate.

The site personnel should use the writing material, which is durable and would not fade over time. Typically, black or blue ball pens are advised for the ease of photocopying. Corrections should be clear with a strikethrough line that does not mask the original writing with initials and date. Original trial documents should never be destroyed.

Documentation should be completed on a real-time basis and should be archived in a manner that allows ready retrieval by authorized personnel for audit or inspection. Secure archival and access control is important to comply with privacy regulations. There should be clarity on personnel who have access to various documents.

Deficiencies in proper documentation arise due to lack of awareness, training, differences in expectation between clinical practice and clinical research, adequate time, manpower and commitment. Systematic lapses lead to obvious questions from an independent observer on accuracy, credibility, and integrity of data. All stakeholders should be sensitive to the overall implications. Periodic verification of site documentation is a routine monitoring responsibility. Monitors play a key role to identify such issues to trigger timely corrective measures. Sponsors may conduct independent audits in critical regulatory submission trials to ensure adequacy, completeness, and accuracy of the trial documentation.

There is a huge momentum in the clinical trial industry to migrate to a paperless environment. It has a direct implication on source documentation at the clinical sites, sponsor locations, and other service providers. While regulatory guidance on this topic is available to some extent, full clarity is lacking at the time of writing this edition. Nonetheless, there is gradual progress in this area. It is common to come across situations of electronic source documentation use at clinical sites, and it is prudent to seek guidance from quality assurance function before allowing such use.

66. Informed consent process

Informed consent is defined in ICH GCP (good clinical practice) as 'a process by which a subject voluntarily confirms his or her willingness to participate in a particular trial, after having been informed of all aspects of the trial that are relevant to the subject's decision to participate. Informed consent is documented by means of a written, signed and dated informed consent form.' A free and fair consent is the foundation of ethical research and GCP.

The consent process for literate adults with sound mental capacity is rather straightforward; however, variations are necessary depending on the profile of research subjects (vulnerability) and disease condition. There are two goals in this process (i) to provide adequate and relevant information about the proposed research to a potential subject (ii) to obtain the consent to participate with full knowledge of the trial and without any influence. The general approach to obtain consent is discussed here; the content of an informed consent form (ICF) has been discussed separately.

The first step of providing information and educating a potential subject begins from the time of the first contact. General high-level information about the proposed research is provided in the initial interaction (e.g. phone call, face-to-face discussion, a proposal by a treating physician or advertisement). If the subject is interested to know more about the proposed research, a detailed discussion follows.

In general, the investigator leads the discussion with the potential subject to obtain consent. Depending on the complexity of the trial, other staff members such as a nurse may assist in the process. All elements in the ICF should be discussed taking sufficient time. The subject should get an opportunity to think through the proposal and ask questions to clarify any aspect of the research before taking a decision. Alternatively, the subject can take home a copy for further reading and discussion with friends, family members or a primary physician. In the next meeting, the subject may ask questions to the investigator to clarify any concerns.

Once the subject is fully satisfied and is willing to take part in the trial, both the subject and the investigator sign the ICF with a date to complete the consenting process. There are usually two copies of the ICF, one stays with the subject and the other with the investigator. The receipt of a copy of ICF should also be documented with the signature of the subject or the legally authorized representative. Typically, the interaction with the investigator and the site staff for ICF discussion is conducted on a one to one basis. However, when multiple subjects are present, information about the study may be provided in a group followed by questions/answer sessions if locally acceptable. In general, some time must be spent in one to one sessions to allow the subjects to clarify any concerns privately. Investigators or site staff may also ask questions to the subjects to assess understanding of the trial.

The latest version of the ICF approved by the ethics committee, (and by the health authority if applicable) in a language which the subject can read and is conversant with, must be used for obtaining consent. Subjects should also have access to the ethics committee to ask questions about the study; typically, the contact details are available in the ICF.

Usually, an impartial witness is present during the consent process to attest that the consent was properly obtained. The provision for an impartial witness should be as per local requirement. As per ICH GCP, an impartial witness is 'a person, who is independent of the trial, who cannot be unfairly influenced by people involved with the trial, who attends the informed consent process if the subject or the subject's legally acceptable representative cannot read, and who reads the informed consent form and any other written information supplied to the subject'.

Some situations are not straightforward, when it involves vulnerable subjects (mentioned below); the ICF process is different to maintain the sanctity of the ethical provision.

- Illiterate subjects
- Children
- Subjects with diminished decision-making capacity
- Pregnant women
- Economically disadvantaged
- Prisoners
- Investigator's own patients
- Students of an investigator

For illiterate subjects, a legally acceptable representative in addition to an impartial witness may be essential. The impartial witness attests that the information in the ICF was accurately explained and was understood by the subject, while the consent is provided by the legally acceptable representative.

For pediatric subjects, assent is taken from the minor subjects after a certain age, while consent is provided by their parents or legal guardians i.e. legally acceptable representative. In some countries, consent of both parents is necessary for the pediatric subjects. In places, where there is a higher rate of separation, it could be problematic if parents have not legally separated and the child does not have a legal custodian. In long duration pediatric trials, subjects may become eligible for assent or consent due to newly attained age; subjects are re-consented with age-appropriate assent or consent accordingly.

Obtaining consent from subjects who have diminished decision-making capacity may involve two stages (i) Evaluation of the mental capacity to determine their capacity to consent (ii) To obtain consent from a legally authorized representative.

US department of health and human services defines legally authorized representative (LAR) as an individual or judicial or other body authorized under applicable law to consent on behalf of a prospective subject to the subject's participation in the procedure(s) involved in the research. When a legally authorized representative is not available for these subjects, other methods are available such as involving ethics committees, caregivers, family members or patient advocates. However, this can be controversial.

For research in a pregnant woman, consent of the pregnant woman and the biological father of the fetus is required if there is any prospect of direct benefit to the fetus from the research except in certain circumstances e.g. the father is incompetent, or the pregnancy resulted from rape.

In situations, where there can be conflicts of interest or obligations of the subjects to an investigator, an independent physician or nurse can witness the process to ensure impartiality and the subjects can be re-contacted later by an independent person to verify willingness. There are circumstances when the ethics committee may waive off requirement of a written consent if it is believed that the research does not compromise the rights and safety of subjects and that the research can't be carried out with this provision.

There could be variations to the requirement as per local regulations of countries and regions and it should be followed. For instance, new regulation in India requires audio/video recording of the informed consent process. Whenever in doubt, a conservative approach should be followed.

Subjects must be asked for a new consent when there is a change in the research procedure, risk-benefit balance, or arrangement, which may affect the decision of already enrolled subjects (or their legally authorized representatives) to continue participation. Examples of such situations are a change of study drug or dose, new clinical procedures that may lead to discomfort, and new safety findings with the drug that alters the risk-benefit profile.

Whenever there is change in the study protocol, availability of new safety data or change in study administrative structure, ICF revision should be considered. The need for re-consent is evaluated by the sponsor and investigator, and the amended ICF needs to be approved by the ethics committee. As subjects have the right to withdraw from the trial anytime, it is not necessary to re-consent subjects for all instances when notification of new information is contemplated. Certain new information such as a change in contact number of the principal investigator, availability of new standard of care or new safety findings can be provided to the subjects in a letter or verbally with appropriate documentation.

Subjects or their legal representatives can withdraw consent to continue participation in the trial at any time. There can be several reasons for consent withdrawal and the subjects have no obligation to cite a reason. From a scientific perspective, it is important to understand if the reason for discontinuation is an adverse event, lack response, or any other concern related to the trial. In general, the reason for trial discontinuation is explored if the subject is willing to share it. In extreme cases, subjects may request to withhold their already collected data from analysis and reporting. It should be considered on a case-by-case basis, and sponsors may refuse to do so depending on the regulations.

There could be a provision for optional procedures (e.g. additional sample collection) in a study and additional consent is taken separately for such procedures. If a subject is not willing to undergo an optional procedure, it does not prevent the subject from continuation in the study; however, that specific procedure would not be performed in that subject. A sample for pharmacogenetic evaluation is often collected in this manner. Subjects may be asked in the ICF to allow long-term storage of back up or leftover samples for future research after protocol specific analysis is complete. Subjects may check tick boxes in the ICF to write down their preference and agreement. Such info can be collected in eCRF to allow sample management accordingly.

Review of the informed consent documents and the process of obtaining consent at the clinical site is a key monitoring activity. The monitors should be sensitive and aware of local requirements to ensure the validity and appropriateness of the consent process and documentation. As such, consent is a key topic from audit and inspection perspective.

67.Subject recruitment and retention

Clinical trials evaluate safety and efficacy of new medicines and are essential component of drug development. Subjects participating in trials may or may not directly benefit from it. For instance, trials evaluating drug-drug interaction in healthy subjects or pharmacokinetics of a drug in subjects with renal failure don't benefit these subjects. Similarly, patients in short-term trials or randomized to placebo arms, may not get a significant direct benefit.

Current ethical principles prohibit any substantial incentive that can potentially induce trial participation (e.g. better patient care or monetary compensation). The reasons why subjects should participate in trials are debatable and is out of the scope for this discussion. After recruitment, retention until study completion is the next big challenge operationally. Subject recruitment and retention are significant issues in any clinical trial and can be potentially derailing.

Several reasons are cited in the literature as barriers to recruitment and retention. Many potential issues can be foreseen at the time of trial planning. A strategy to overcome the barriers should be worked out with inputs from the clinical sites and it should be implemented from the start. Once the trial begins, unforeseen issues should be promptly addressed.

Here are the four categories of reasons cited as barriers to recruitment:

Subject related:

- Lack of awareness of clinical trials
- Lack of knowledge on trials conducted in the locality
- Content with the available therapies
- Fear, distrust, and suspicion about research
- Inconvenience of participation (time, extra visits, extra procedures, loss of working days, etc)
- Negative influence of friends, family members and primary physician
- Education level (well educated people are more likely to participate)
- Disease severity (more symptomatic subjects are less likely to participate)
- Language barriers
- Minority population category in the society (less likely to participate)
- Cultural belief against modern medicine
- Negative influence of media
- Inadequate compensation
- Conflicts with health or life insurance terms/conditions due to participation

Investigator related:

- Lack of time due to clinical workload

- Lack of interest in clinical research due to extra activity
- Underestimation of involvement (which leads to demotivation later)
- Lack of conviction on the trial objective
- Belief that standard therapy has better efficacy than the experimental therapy
- Safety concerns with the experimental therapy
- Absence of referring primary physicians
- Inadequate financial incentive
- Unfriendly hospital settings or society for clinical research
- Competing trials at the clinical site leading to lack of motivation
- Fear of the unknown

Protocol related:
- Narrow entry criteria
- Complex study designs, intensive or invasive study procedures, lengthy trials, frequent visit schedules
- Treatment protocols grossly different to standard of medical care in the locality
- Placebo controlled trials

Others:

- Inappropriate choice of investigators
- Lack of key opinion leader (KOL) endorsement for the trial
- Reputation of the sponsor or the contract research organization (CRO)

Here are few reasons cited as barriers to retention of subjects until trial completion:

- Inadequate informed consent form (ICF) discussion with the trial subjects
- Trial subjects without adequate knowledge about their responsibilities, study procedures, visits, etc.
- Lack of proper attention at the time of visits from the investigator/site staff and long waiting period

- Lack of active involvement of the investigators (delegation of research activities to study coordinator)
- Adverse events
- Lack of response from study medication or placebo (expectations not met)
- Loss of enthusiasm in long duration trials
- Lack of follow up and encouragement from the site

The above reasons are well known among operation experts and are taken into consideration while planning a trial. Many of the issues listed here are subjective, relative and may vary depending on the context. Some of these can be addressed through proper strategies and swift interventions, while others can be inherent to a particular trial and may not be amenable to easy resolution. Trials in healthy subjects are a bit different from trials in patient subjects and many of the issues discussed above may not be applicable.

A flexible and practical protocol is a good starting point for a successful trial conduct. Protocol development should consider the study objectives, clinical practice standards, feasibility, minimization of a burden to subjects, risk-benefits, and many other practical aspects. Prior experience with similar trials or any insights from literature is helpful. Countries and sites should be carefully chosen considering the prevalence of such disease, similar trial experience, disease pattern, any competitive trials, practice standards, and so on. The input of the investigators in trial planning may be useful; however, may not be so easy to obtain.

The simple arithmetic of planning a higher number of sites for a trial with large sample size is a reasonable approach. Specialized centers may be worth a try, in the context of complex trials. Clinical sites can maximize recruitment efforts by maintaining a database of patients, pre-screening of patients in the outpatient department, arranging referrals from fellow physicians or general practitioners, timely advertisements, meticulous review of the protocol and timely feedback to the sponsor.

Role of careful ICF discussion to the success of recruitment and retention cannot be overemphasized. If the subjects understand the proposed contribution of the trial, their own responsibility, study procedures, foreseen inconveniences, risks, their alternatives as well as have an opportunity to clarify their concerns or consult any other person before taking the decision to participate, the likelihood of discontinuation in the course of the trial would be minimal. Any form of influence is not only unethical but also counterproductive leading to future discontinuation.

Continuous engagement with the investigators during trial conduct through regular meetings, periodic updates, solicitation of feedbacks on difficulties in recruitment or trial conduct, facilitation of best practice sharing between investigators are usually productive. Timely review of subject data on screen failures, trial noncompliance, and withdrawals may give valuable insights. Sites should be encouraged to discuss proactively the issues with the sponsor for any potential solutions. Careful selection of subjects, adequate counselling, and close follow up are tested methods of better compliance.

Despite adequate planning, there may be poor recruitment and retention due to issues that are only evident as the trial progresses. A pragmatic analysis of reasons and trends from various sites should be performed in an open mind. It is important to consider any inherent flaw in the trial protocol if there are similar issues from several sites. If certain sites are able to run the trial successfully, there may be other site-specific issues to deal with. Timely amendment of the protocol may salvage the situation early in the trial. Aggressive follow-up and engagements with the sites are the usual approaches. Compensation to investigators and trial subjects may be revised if perceived as a concern. Best practices of successful sites may be tried at other sites if possible. Closing or de-prioritizing non-performing sites as well as activation of backup or new sites are in general the last resort measures.

During the trial setup phase, it is important to have a discussion on recruitment and retention with site personnel e.g. strategies on recruitment, the source of recruitment, advertisements, potential foreseen challenges, strategies on retention or subject engagement. It is a good practice to orient the sites to plan and document the plans as necessary. It is important to ensure the sites have budget covered for such activities. Typically, an advertisement for recruitment or any retention strategy (e.g. customary gifts) needs approval by EC.

Recruitment and retention have serious bearing beyond the study operations such as financial implications, prompt availability of data for regulatory submission, key decisions, or timelines of downstream activities. Key stakeholders must be made aware of the circumstances while dealing with such demanding situations for any adjustments or any mitigation of dependent activities.

68. Trial subject management

Trial subject management is the most demanding activity at a clinical site. The broader motivations in the context of subject management are adherence to ethical principles, protocol compliance and ensuring subject safety while achieving the trial goal of answering scientific questions. Subjects remain in the purview of the investigator and the clinical site team from the time of initial contact until safe discharge from a trial. Besides the routine efforts on recruitment and retention, certain general aspects are important considerations while dealing with trial subjects.

There is a subtle difference in the management of patients in clinical trials vs. that in routine medical care. Subjects in clinical trials have different expectations as they have more responsibilities and obligations in comparison to general patients. Similarly, expectations of the investigators from trial subjects are also different. Healthy subjects taking part in clinical trials in an entirely different context.

Clinical pharmacology units dealing with healthy subject trials have a database of potential participants and many of them periodically participate in such trials. New subjects come in through contacts, word of mouth and advertisements. In patient trials, the subjects are recruited from investigator's own practice patient pool or referrals from other physicians. Some investigators, who are routinely involved in clinical research, may have databases of patients (typically having chronic illnesses). Patients may directly approach investigators once aware of the trials with an intention to get access to innovative treatment options not yet available in the market.

Subject's identity should be established through appropriate documents and identification marks. When there are multiple subjects at the site (e.g. domiciled stay in healthy subject trials) identity cards or wrist tags may be used to identify subjects. Biometrics systems (e.g. use of fingerprints for identity) are increasingly used as an alternative. Strategies to prevent cross participation are important, especially in healthy volunteer trials. IT-enabled biometric systems in collaboration with other research centers are in use in some places.

Trial subjects should be easily accessible by telephone or email. It is essential for the sites to be able to communicate readily with subjects for follow-up, reminder, safety enquiry or to provide trial-related information. In certain trials, mobile devices are provided to trial subjects that can measure body function, serve as an electronic diary, or trigger reminder. Subjects should be encouraged to be in touch with the investigator or a representative for any medical or other trial-related problems. Each subject should be explained about his/her visit plan in the trial. At each visit, the plan for the next visit should be discussed. Typically, it is normal practice for the clinical sites to remind subjects over the phone about an upcoming visit.

It is important to pay due attention to trial subjects during every visit and interaction. Trial visits should be scheduled as per the convenience of the subjects as possible and waiting period at the site should be minimized. It is a good practice for site staff to accompany the subjects to make them comfortable while at the trial site. The investigator and the study coordinator should try to know the trial subjects personally. Subjects typically appreciate when investigators spend some time with them at each visit even though it may not be needed. While hospitalized for trial procedures, subjects may be encouraged to engage in acceptable recreational activities. Subjects should be periodically reminded about their responsibilities and duly appreciated for their contribution.

It is not unusual to have delicate situations such as subjects experiencing serious trial-related adverse events, opting to discontinue from a trial, noncompliance to trial protocol, seeking compensation for trial-related adverse events, dissatisfied with response to trial treatment, burdened by trial requirements, losing enthusiasm to continue in the trial, unhappy with site personnel, disturbed by rumours or negative opinions about the trial, etc.

Such situations should be expected, and site staff should be trained to handle that professionally with compassion and fairness. Sponsor organizations should be made aware of such situations on a real-time basis. Rarely, such situations may get out of control and become media stories or social media talking points. Media training is typically provided to investigators in field trials of vaccines to manage rumors spreading in the community. Investigators have the responsibility to act in the interest of trial subjects, and sponsors should have a pragmatic approach to facilitate resolution of issues as acceptable locally. Local ethics committee may be consulted if necessary for guidance.

69.Center number, subject number, randomization, and treatment allocation

Unique identification is crucial to accurately link treatments and data to individual subjects in a clinical trial. Hence, subjects, centers, treatments, medications, and sequence of treatments are uniquely numbered. This is also conducive to data management, statistical analysis and reporting in an electronic environment. Randomization minimizes bias in treatment allocation to individual subjects. Typically, organizations have standard operating procedures on such processes and the convention is clarified in the protocol. A set of conventions is discussed here as examples for understanding and organizations may have their conventions.

All clinical sites (centers) are numbered regardless of the total number of sites in a trial. It can be started with 1 and then in increasing order as 2,3, and so on or started with another number such as 101 and then in the increasing order as 102, 103, and so on. For multi-country trials, each country may be identified by a code (e.g. first three letters of a country) or a number. Regions with a similar standard of care may have unique codes or numbers to facilitate analysis. The center number is typically a combination of these codes and numbers as discussed above.

Subjects are assigned screening or enrolment numbers once they consent to participate and are ready for screening. It can be a combination of the center number and another number in an ascending order. The determinant of the other number can be the time of informed consent. For instance, if the first subject is numbered 01, the second subject should be numbered 02 and so on. The screening number once assigned is not reused by the center, so that it remains unique in the trial.

Once a subject is eligible to receive trial intervention after a successful screening, a randomization number or treatment number is assigned. 'Treatment number' and 'randomization number' are synonymous. Typically, the term 'randomization number' is used where a randomization process is involved; in nonrandomized trials, the term 'treatment number' is used. This number is provisional until a subject commences treatment. If the subject cannot receive the trial treatment after assignment of a randomization or treatment number, another subject can be assigned that number. However, it must be documented appropriately. Like screening numbers, treatment or randomization numbers are also assigned sequentially in ascending order.

The clinical sites maintain records linking the screening numbers with the randomization or treatment numbers for tracking. It is usually reviewed and verified by the field monitor for accuracy. Either the screening number or the treatment/randomization number can be considered as the actual subject number in a trial and is used for identification of individual subjects throughout the trial e.g. to identify biological samples. This arrangement of separate screening and randomization/treatment numbers are common when a specific set of randomization/treatment numbers have been supplied to sites for use. In central randomization with interactive technologies, subjects commonly have just one unique number assigned at the time of enrolment for use throughout the trial i.e. there are no different screening and randomization/treatment number.

Randomization is the process of allocation of treatment arms or sequences (in crossover design) to trial subjects. It is only applicable in situations where there is more than one treatment to choose. Thus, trials with only one treatment have no need for randomization to allocate treatment. In randomized trials, once treatment allocation is determined through randomization, it is typically concealed to a certain extent through the process of blinding. Randomization ensures that the investigators have no control over treatment selection for individual subjects. The operational process of randomization and subsequent treatment allocation varies depending on the number of centers, the number of treatment arms, study design, blinding requirement, IP packaging and IP supply plan.

A few scenarios are discussed here for understanding:

Single center studies:

A. Open label randomized trial with bulk investigational product (IP) supply: A randomization list containing subject numbers in increasing order and treatment allocations against it is provided to the site pharmacist. Individual subject specific medication packs are prepared at the site and dispensed or directly administered according to the treatment allocation. The randomization list remains confidential with the pharmacist until treatment is initiated.

B. Single blind (subject is blind to treatment), randomized trial with bulk IP supply: The process remains as in (A), except that the treatment in different arms should look similar. Information about treatment allocation is not disclosed to subjects until database lock. Investigator or study personnel have access to this information.

C. Double blind (both investigator and subject are blind to treatment), randomized trial with bulk IP supply: A pharmacist (called unblinded pharmacist) at the site receives the randomization list and prepares as well as dispenses treatments accordingly. The unblinded pharmacist is not involved in drug administration. Another pharmacist (called blinded pharmacist) without any knowledge to treatment allocation handles drug administration. No other trial team members get access to information on treatment allocation; confidentiality is maintained until database lock.

D. Open-label or blinded, randomized trial with IP supply as subject packs: IP is supplied pre-packaged for individual subjects to the pharmacist. Once a subject is eligible for treatment in the trial and gets a randomization number, the corresponding IP pack is dispensed. Treatment allocation information is not available at the site in case of double-blind trials. However, this information is provided to the pharmacist in case of single-blind (where subjects are only blinded) and open-label trials.

Multi-center trials:

The randomization process is a bit different due to multiple sites in the trial. To circumvent the situation, site-specific randomization lists can be supplied to the sites. For example, if 100 subjects were to be recruited in a trial from 10 sites, each site could be supplied 10 numbers. However, recruitment across sites is often not uniform, and typically, there is competitive recruitment. Alternatively, randomization information for few subjects can be supplied to the sites to begin recruitment. Randomization information for more subjects could be supplied later depending on recruitment progress. Randomization information can be retrieved from non-recruiting centers to be resupplied to other centers. However, this process may have logistic challenges.

In another approach, randomization lists can be prepared for a higher number of subjects for each site (e.g. 20 numbers for each site and 200 in total for a sample size of 100) with a presumption that recruitment at any site would not be more than this. Central supervision is essential in this approach to ensure that recruitment across sites doesn't exceed the sample size.

The commonly used strategy in multicenter trials is central randomization, although it may not be cost-effective in smaller trials. Central randomization could be a manual email based system, where randomization information is provided through emails upon request or through interactive response technology (IRT). In the former, the sites are pre-supplied with information linking the randomization number to treatment allocation. A manual email based system has logistics issues as it requires human intervention on demand and may be feasible in trials with few centers. Interactive response technology (IRT) is suitable for larger trials.

Interactive Response Technology: IRT can be voice-based i.e. IVRS (Interactive Voice Response System) or web-based i.e. IWRS (Interactive Web Response Technology). In IVRS, the authorized site personnel call a number and input required information using telephone keypad in response to prompted pre-recorded simple questions. Once correct information is inputted, the necessary information is given out or sent through emails. The process could be assisted via a call center. IWRS works in a similar fashion through a specially designed web portal. Besides randomization and treatment allocation, IRT is also helpful in other aspects of enrolment and drug supply.

The information retrieved from IRT depends on the nature of packaging and IP supply plan. It could be treatment allocation (i.e. treatment X or Y) in case of bulk IP supply where the IP has not been packaged as individual subject packs or medication pack numbers if IP has been packaged as individual subject packs.

Most patient trials have provision for home treatment (i.e. subjects are dispensed IP to take at home). In such trials, subject-specific medication packs can be provided to the sites or prepared at the sites. The process is similar to scenario A, when bulk IP is supplied instead of patient packs in open-label trials. In blinded trials, patient packs need to look similar (along with the medication inside) for effective blinding and the process may be as in scenario B or C. In double-blind trials, when unblinded pharmacist arrangement is not possible, identical looking patient packs need to be supplied to the site.

Typically, a higher number of patient packs is supplied to sites and IRT may be programmed with a higher number of randomization numbers, as recruitment is not uniform across the sites. It must be monitored that the total recruitment across the sites doesn't exceed the planned sample size, and it could be controlled by IRT.

Significant dropout and withdrawals are generally managed through planned over recruitment. Sometimes, subject replacement is an option, typically in healthy subject trials. In such cases, a second set of randomization numbers is assigned to the replaced subjects. For each withdrawn subject, a new subject is randomized in the study. The randomization needs to be planned in such a manner that the treatment allocation of a replaced subject is same as that of a withdrawn subject.

When the trial is such that a differential response to the treatments is expected in subgroups of the population (e.g. different classes of heart failure, age-groups, and regions), stratified randomization is considered to balance the number of subjects from each sub-group in different treatment arms. It ensures balanced representation of different sub-groups in each arm to understand effects in different sub-groups of population and balanced representation of each arm within each subgroup to allow a proper comparison. Operationally, it could be 'fixed number stratification' so that a predetermined number of subjects of each sub-group are in each arm. The other option is 'flexible number stratified randomization' with a minimum target for each sub-group. It is also important to have a similar number of subjects in different treatment arms at any given time, and block randomization is used for this.

Besides treatment allocation, randomization may be required for selection of a subset of subjects for additional evaluation or long-term follow up. In such cases, randomization is still required even if the trial has only one treatment arm. It is necessary to inform subjects through ICF about such random allocation.

Randomization information is confidential in nature and confidentiality is maintained through agreements, secured emails, login credentials in electronic systems, security questions in case of IRT and provision of independent study team members.

70.Blinding in clinical trial conduct

Sponsor, investigator or other study personnel may have certain perceptions about the investigational treatments in a trial. This may potentially influence the trial conduct, the manner of data generation, analysis and interpretation. Blinding and randomization are two established ways to reduce such bias in clinical trials. Blinding is a set of steps followed to conceal treatment allocation information from trial subjects, investigators or other study personnel. The modality and extent of blinding depend on the objective and nature of assessments in a trial. Blinding may be restricted to one of the parties (trial subjects, investigators and other study personnel e.g. pharmacist, laboratory technician) or multiple parties in a trial.

Blinding prevents any bias (about an investigational treatment) to influence the evaluation of endpoints or data interpretation (e.g. adverse events). Blinding is particularly important in trials with subjective endpoints, which are evaluated by the investigators (e.g. physician reported outcome score, radiological assessment). However, objective endpoints (e.g. plasma level of a drug or a laboratory parameter) are not affected by prior knowledge of treatment allocation. However, certain decisions in any trial (e.g. evaluation of the severity of adverse events or subject withdrawal for lack of response) have subjective component and hence, blinding is an important consideration.

On the other hand, randomization is a process of random assignment of investigational treatments to trial subjects in such a way that the investigator or other study personnel have no influence on treatment allocation and hence, prevents selection bias. Randomization has been discussed in another section of this book.

The blinding process should be clearly outlined in the protocol or in another document. It should include the extent of blinding, rationale, the methods to be followed to maintain blinding, personnel who would be blinded, and duration of blinding as well as conditions when blinding may be broken and the method. Arrangement for blinding is one of the key considerations in trial planning operationally.

In a typical double-blind trial, the sponsor's medical monitor, investigators, trial subjects and the study personnel at the clinical sites remain blinded to treatment allocation until database lock. Certain study personnel (e.g. a pharmacist, an independent investigator) who are not involved in any routine study activity may have access to treatment allocation (e.g. drug dispensing, safety evaluation) as required. An independent study monitor reviews drug dispensing which requires knowledge of treatment allocation and is not involved in routine monitoring. Generally, the randomization scheme with treatment allocation information is made available to the trial team after database lock.

Treatment allocation is necessary after database lock to identify treatment groups for statistical analysis. Typically, the randomization scheme release is requested by the trial team with a copy of database lock memo.

The similar appearance of drug products in different treatment arms is essential for effective blinding. This may not be feasible all the time or can be logistically prohibitive. Modification to comparator drug product of a competitor company is generally difficult. Blinding in such situations can be achieved through a double dummy technique if matching placebos to the active treatments are available. For instance, in a study with two active treatment arms, a subject would receive an active pill and a matching placebo of the other active comparator pill in each arm.

Over-encapsulation of a comparator drug to look like an investigational drug is possible in certain instances. In extreme cases, physically blinding the subjects with sleeping masks may be feasible in a setting where supervised drug administration is planned. For injectable preparations, which could be of different color, use of syringe sheaths, sticker around syringes or administration behind a privacy film has been tried.

The unique effect of study treatments on body physiology can be a hindrance to effective blinding. For instance, certain drugs may cause discoloration of urine leading to treatment identification. Trial subjects may measure common parameters such as blood pressure out of curiosity. Laboratory data of subjects may be suggestive of certain treatments due to unique effects.

Proper mechanisms should be set up at the site, so that, investigators may remain blinded while the safety of the subjects is not compromised. Certain laboratory parameters may be withheld from routine reporting unless a trigger level is breached; alternatively, independent investigators (not involved in routine study activities) can be engaged to assess sensitive parameters and respond appropriately.

Trial subjects must be informed about the blinding requirements in a study. The extent of study information provided in the informed consent form to subjects should be carefully determined. Placebo run-in period is especially tricky, as subjects may not comply with such provisions leading to bias in assessment. In such trials, subjects may be informed about possible placebo use in the trial without specifying the exact period of use.

Data management of blinded data requires meticulous planning of database design, data entry, and review. Independent study team members can be involved at each of these steps. Certain techniques such as masking of certain data or scrambling of subject numbers and visits are helpful at the time of data review to maintain blinding.

Identification of treatment allocation may be required in exceptional circumstances to manage adverse events in a trial. A set of emergency code breaks is usually provided to the investigator to manage these situations. The code breaks may be stored at the pharmacy, emergency facility or with the investigator depending on local practice or country regulation. In large trials, this is typically managed through IRT portals (Interactive Response Technology) where investigators or authorized personnel can input specific information to obtain the treatment allocation.

Any code break must be documented along with time and rationale. Knowledge of the treatment allocation may not be useful for adverse event management in all situations due to lack of an antidote or generic approach to medical management of the AE. Sponsor's medical monitor may be consulted for the need for unblinding to manage a medical emergency. Any unblinding event should be brought to the attention of the monitor and sponsor to assess the impact. The IRT portals can be programmed to send alerts to relevant personnel in the trial once a subject is unblinded. The protocol should generally indicate how to manage subjects once unblinded by the investigator; else, it may be decided on a case by case basis.

Blinding considerations require detailed planning involving various functions involved in clinical trials such as drug supply, statistics, clinical laboratory, data management, medical monitoring, clinical operations as well as clinical site personnel. Planning is necessary early on, as some of the elements may be time-consuming such as manufacturing or sourcing an identical-looking placebo. Any specific requirements from the sites should be part of feasibility evaluation. Due to the sensitivity of the topic from a regulatory perspective, most organizations have detailed SOPs on various aspects of blinding in clinical trials. When blinded and unblinded team arrangement is necessary, a communication flow is crucial, and it needs to be defined.

Accidental code breaks in trial by the sponsor or the clinical site staffs is not uncommon. One of the common sources of accidental unblinding is inadvertent sharing of IRT reports containing treatment allocation information through email. Minimizing both access and duration of such access to unblinded information is generally helpful. An access controlled portal may be used for communication between unblinded team members. Action plans should be available to deal with such situations in consultation with quality assurance group.

71. Investigational product dispensing, administration, and reconciliation

Investigational product (IP) handling is one of the most sensitive activities in a clinical trial from a regulatory perspective. Generally, IP is supplied to the clinical site by the sponsor or bought from the market by the investigator. At the clinical site, IP remains in custody of the investigator, study pharmacist or any other authorized person in appropriate conditions until it is dispensed, returned or destroyed with full accountability.

IP is often dispensed to trial subjects for self-administration at home; alternatively, IP may be administered to subjects by study personnel at the clinical facility. After treatment phase is over or periodically as necessary, all unused IP is retrieved from the subjects by the investigator or study staff and is kept in custody of the pharmacist or any other authorized personnel. During a trial, appropriate documentation is maintained on dispensing, drug administration (if administered at the clinical facility), return of unused IP and reconciliation. Finally, the IP may be returned to sponsor for destruction (or another purpose) or destroyed by the site after written authorization from a sponsor. In general, IP meant for use in a clinical trial is not used for any other purpose or in another clinical trial.

IP may be supplied to the clinical site as bulk (to be packaged for individual subjects) or as subject-specific packs. Few factors for consideration to supply IP as bulk or individual patient packs are (i) domiciled or outpatient drug administration (ii) facility for blinding (iii) scale of the trial (number of subjects, sites and duration) (iv) facility for dispensing (v) country regulation (vi) randomization and blinding requirement.

When IP is supplied as bulk, the pharmacist prepares subject specific packs and dispenses according to randomization scheme or treatment allocation. In a blinded trial, an unblinded pharmacist, who has knowledge of treatment allocation and is not involved in any other trial activity, dispenses IP to the trial team (for supervised administration) or to the subjects. On the other hand, IP supplied as subject pack is directly dispensed as per randomization scheme. In such cases, blinding is typically implemented centrally, and the sites remain blinded to treatment allocation. Depending on the arrangement for randomization and blinding, this step may be performed in many ways and has been discussed separately.

Dispensing and administration of IP is governed by local (country/state) regulations. For instance, in certain countries, GMP (Good Manufacturing Practice) facility may be required for dispensing unit doses from bulk medication or reconstituting a powder form to liquid formulation (if the primary packing is manipulated). It may not be required elsewhere. Such operational aspects should be enquired during site selection.

It is a common practice to prepare unit doses for individual subjects in clinical pharmacology units. The unit doses are placed in small containers or plastic pouches and labelled. A similar process may be followed in hospitals where supervised drug administration has been planned to ensure compliance. Unit dose preparation from bulk supplies is a critical and confidential step in blinded trials. Quality control measures should be in place to ensure the accuracy of drug, dose, and treatment allocation. IP dispensing is typically monitored to a certain extent by a field monitor in view of the importance of that step. For complex unit dose preparations (e.g. injectable, inhalational, intraocular, reconstitution of powder to liquid, etc), a detailed manual (or video) is generally prepared for the ease of understanding and clarity; the site staff should be explicitly trained on it.

Details of IP administration are recorded in subject files or other source documents. When drug administration is at the site, study staff can document it themselves. Mouth check after oral drug administration ensures that the drug was swallowed by the subject and is commonly necessary for clinical pharmacology studies. For self- administration outside the trial facility, subjects may be provided with a diary record certain basic information (e.g. time, fasting/fed state, and dose) to document compliance. It is also important to document any deviation from planned drug administration. Such information is typically collected in the eCRF.

Here are few considerations to determine the need for supervised administration at the study centers (i) compliance is critical (ii) complex preparation and administration steps involved (iii) immediate safety concerns where observation is warranted (iv) blinding considerations. Newer technologies are available to remind subjects for drug intake or notify clinical sites of drug intake remotely. Such technologies work through mobile networks and help to enhance compliance and automatic documentation of drug administration.

Special attention is required in trials with pharmacokinetics as the primary endpoint. For oral drug administration, the volume of water, subject posture, fasting/fed condition, and food intake are standardized as these may affect pharmacokinetics. Clear instruction in detail should be provided for drug administration (e.g. if a tablet needs to be chewed or directly swallowed). Certain drug administration requires familiarization and practice by the subjects as well as site staff (e.g. inhalational drugs). Practice sessions with placebo may be performed before randomization and demonstration of acceptable use may be an entry criterion.

Clinical sites maintain documentation of IP received, dispensed to subjects, returned from subjects, destroyed, returned to sponsor and any archival as retention samples. Reconciliation and accountability of IP supply, dispensing or return need to be carried out on an ongoing basis or at least at the trial closeout. It prevents any misuse of IP meant for clinical trials and ensures controlled handling. At the end of a trial, remaining IP need to be destroyed or returned to the sponsor, and this step must be documented. Electronic method is increasingly in use to automate many of these steps.

72.Biological sample handling at the trial site

Results of biological sample analysis can be impacted by deviations to collection time, processing, storage, transport, and analysis. In a clinical trial, certain samples may be analyzed at the local laboratory while others are shipped to one or more central laboratories. The complexity increases when there are samples with differing requirements and involvement of multiple laboratories. Planning during protocol development has been discussed in another section; the focus here is on sample handling at the trial site.

Biological samples may be blood, urine, stool, tissue, synovial fluid, cerebrospinal fluid, peritoneal fluid, semen, and so on. Procedures for collection, processing, storage, and shipment are detailed in the protocol or in a laboratory manual. In addition, sites may have standard operating procedures (SOP) on these procedures. Sponsors and clinical sites need to ensure availability of necessary instruments, accessories, personnel, and storage conditions before enrolling subjects. Sponsors should ensure appropriate training of the site personnel. A dry run at the clinical site before the actual trial is helpful to identify potential problems. Back up arrangements are important, as there may be little flexibility when subjects are at the sites.

Coordination among different site personnel is important for the seamless flow of activities. Subject preparation may be essential prior to sample collection. Certain samples need to be collected in fasting condition, others after a period of rest and so on. This should be discussed with the subjects as part of the consent process but also reminded prior to each visit.

Samples should be labelled appropriately with necessary information such as trial number, center number, subject number, sample type, sample number, the name of an analyte, collection time or as otherwise specified in the protocol/laboratory manual. Typically, empty sample containers are pre-labelled before sample collection. Various labelling techniques such as barcode labels and duplicate tear off labels (for subject files, shipping invoice, and the tubes) are used for precise traceability. Once collected, samples should be swiftly processed and stored as per instructions. In certain trials, samples are collected in duplicate as a contingency measure. Typically, these duplicate (back up) samples are only shipped after the primary aliquots reach the labs; both must not be shipped together.

Typically, aliquots of samples are arranged in a specific order in cryoboxes prior to storage to allow easy identification and retrieval during subsequent handling and analysis. The cryoboxes should also be labelled appropriately. All samples from one subject may be analyzed together while in other situations, samples for a visit for all subjects are analyzed together. In large trials with a significant volume of samples and with increased reliance on barcode labels, manual identification of a set of samples could be difficult due to storage at extreme temperatures. Inventory management techniques are important both at the site and at the central laboratory. It should be considered and planned appropriately. Often, prioritization of some sample analysis is necessary.

Biological samples are typically shipped in a temperature-controlled environment, although some samples can be shipped in ambient conditions. Temperature probes with data loggers should be included in the shipments accordingly. For inter country shipments, the import/export licenses must be ready before trial initiation. During shipment, the concerned parties should be informed appropriately, so that, samples remain attended during transportation. Holiday schedules of the shipment agency and recipient laboratories should be considered while planning subject visits. Frozen samples are typically shipped in dry ice or liquid nitrogen. Generally, the shipping agency makes such arrangements and must be confirmed prior to subject visits.

Each step involved in sample handling from collection until shipment and receipt are documented. Time of sample collection, processing, storage, and further shipment of each sample is recorded in specially designed logbooks or forms. Any problem or deviation in any of the steps is documented appropriately. The temperature of the storage conditions at the clinical site must be maintained and documented on an ongoing basis. Generally, the freezers or the walk-in cold rooms would have inbuilt monitors to measure and record temperature. Increasing many of such documentation have been automated due to use of electronic methods e.g. electronic requisition forms.

Samples are shipped along with an invoice with details of the samples and storage conditions for reference. The recipient laboratory would typically perform a reconciliation of the samples received against the invoice. Generally, the transport condition is reviewed at the laboratory while receiving the samples. Records of shipment including temperature logs are filed in the trial master file for archival. Further documentation of sample handling until the analysis is maintained at the laboratory.

Any specific requirements such as expedited shipment, additional labelling elements, and specific processing steps must be clarified explicitly in the protocol or lab manual as well as reviewed and reminded by the trial monitors. Swift feedback from the central labs on received sample quality or any documentation issues should be communicated the site to correct any errors especially in the initial phase of trials. In long-term trials, trial-specific steps may be omitted inadvertently with the passage of time and change in site personnel. Trial monitors should proactively reinforce the importance of such steps periodically.

Despite apparent meticulous planning, typical issues at the sites are shippers not arriving in time, lack of capacity in freezers, non-availability of centrifuge, power outage, omission of processing steps, incomplete documentation, inadequate sample volume collection, subject refusing blood sample, inadequate subject preparation, failure to order resupply of lab accessories, use of wrong tubes, failure to place temperature probes in shipments, etc. While it may be difficult to totally avoid some of these practical issues, mitigation steps should be taken swiftly to minimize the impact.

73.Adverse event management

An adverse event (AE) is defined as an unfavorable and unintended sign, symptom, or disease temporally associated with the use of a medicinal (investigational) product, irrespective of its relation to the medicinal (investigational) product. Worsening of existing medical conditions and laboratory abnormalities, which are clinically significant or need medical intervention are also termed as AEs. An AE may or may not be related to the investigational product (IP). When a causal relationship is a reasonable possibility i.e. the relationship cannot be ruled out, it is termed as adverse drug reaction (ADR).

Typically, safety information is collected, reported, and interpreted as per the protocol, standard operating procedures (SOP) and regulations. The potential AEs with an IP are determined based on its pharmacological class, preclinical studies in animals or in vitro systems as well as experience in humans. Trials are designed to assess the occurrence of specific anticipated AEs as well as other AEs not anticipated as a generic approach. The assessment of AEs may require specific assessments (e.g. ECG, radiological tests, lab tests, etc) at specific time points after IP administration. With a gain of substantial experience with the IP, AEs observed but not anticipated earlier are added to the safety profile while AEs anticipated earlier may be downgraded if not observed in clinical trials. Pharmacovigilance function plays a key role in this process.

AEs may be expected or unexpected and may or may not be related to the trial IPs. One of the key objectives of any clinical trial is to evaluate the safety of the IP and therefore, any AE in a trial is reviewed carefully. Generally, AE is enquired through open questions and leading questions such as 'did you have a headache' are avoided. Subjects are encouraged to contact the site in case of any AE or events leading medical consultations or emergency room visits as soon as possible. In specific situations such as vaccine trials, it is common to solicit information about injection site reactions, temperature and certain systemic symptoms; these are called solicited AEs. Typically, a diary card is provided to complete daily for specific durations post vaccination.

Safety of the trial subjects is of utmost importance and remains primarily with the investigator, while the sponsor has the ultimate responsibility. The ethics committee (EC) and health authority (HA) have a supervisory role from a governance perspective.

Relationship with the IP is reported as suspected (certain/definitely related/ probable/likely related/ possibly related), non-suspected (not suspected or unlikely related) or not applicable. Establishing the relationship or causality of an AE to an IP is a complex process and beyond the scope of this discussion. Biological plausibility, preclinical signals, prior experience, temporal association, disproportionate occurrence in comparison to placebo arms or general population, subsidence after discontinuation and resumption after re-administration are the key considerations to claim or refute causality. The investigator is responsible for causality assessment of individual AEs in a trial.

To bring a certain degree of standardization, all AEs in a particular timeframe of the trial are collected and subjected to causality assessment. The timeframe may be from the moment of the first dose of the IP until a reasonable time after the last dose or specific time intervals after each dose e.g. in vaccine trials.

Sometimes, all AEs from the point of enrolment (signing the consent) are collected and evaluated.

Clear guidance needs to be provided in the protocol and eCRF completion guidelines to define and appropriately report AEs; considerable time is spent in capturing such data accurately. For reporting purposes, one medical event is considered as one medical concept and hence, one AE term is used to report one AE; the diagnosis of an event rather each symptom/sign is reported unless no diagnosis could be made. Pre-existing conditions, pre-planned surgeries, or procedures scheduled prior to trial participation, elective surgeries or procedures during the trial where there is no change in medical conditions as well as diagnostic procedures need not be reported as AEs. However, any complications arising from surgeries or procedures qualify as AEs.

Description of the AE, time of occurrence and resolution, severity, action taken, and opinion on relationship to the IP are typically reported in the case report form (CRF). If an AE was not resolved at the last evaluation, it should also be reported (e.g. continuing at last visit). Once an AE is detected, it is followed up until resolution or when deemed permanent. The follow up may happen in subsequent scheduled or unscheduled visits. Any change in severity noted at the follow-up visits is documented. The actions taken for an AE can be: (a) observation only (i.e. no action taken), (b) study treatment interruption or modification, (c) permanent discontinuation of study treatment, (d) drug or nondrug therapy administration, (e) hospitalization or prolongation of hospitalization.

Severities of the AE are described as mild, moderate, and severe (including life-threatening and death) or in the CTCAE grade. It is important to provide guidance on different criteria with examples for clarity. As AE severity is expected to change over time, the event is generally captured once with the maximum severity. The AE is assessed for the fulfilment of serious adverse event (SAE) criteria. An AE is classified as a SAE fulfilling any of the following criteria: (a) results in death, (b) life-threatening,

(c) requires inpatient hospitalization or prolongation of existing hospitalization, (d) results in persistent or significant disability/incapacity (e) is a congenital anomaly/birth defect (f) is a medically important event or reaction. Death per se is not an AE but the outcome and the condition(s) leading to death needs to be reported as AE.

Reporting responsibilities in case of an SAE should be kept in mind. The investigator must report the SAE to the sponsor within 24 hours of learning its occurrence unless the protocol prescribes another reporting timeframe. The investigator also has the responsibility of notifying such events to the EC, whereas, it's the sponsor's responsibility to notify the SAEs to the HA and other investigators. The SAEs are reported to other investigators in the form of investigator notification (IN). Other investigators, in turn, report it to their respective ECs.

Reporting timeframe and need for expedited reporting also depend on the country regulation, expectedness of the SAE and relationship to the IP. The investigator's brochure or the product monograph usually lists down expected AEs, which is called reference safety information (RSI). Any AE which is not listed in the RSI is considered unexpected. At periodic intervals, aggregate reports of SAEs/AEs from all trials with an IP along with risk-benefit assessment are distributed to all the investigators, HAs and ECs depending on the local regulations.

In view of the importance of SAE reporting for subject safety and regulatory compliance, investigators and site staff are trained on reporting requirement prior to the start of the trial and at periodic intervals as necessary. Investigators and site personnel are specifically trained on the safety of the investigational products including expected AEs, specific AEs of interest, reporting timeframes, trial-specific modality of reporting, SAE forms and its data fields, managing situations requiring treatment code break, common errors and specific care to minimize queries. Typical errors observed are causality assessments not made by the investigator, incomplete relevant information on the SAE form, failure to provide follow-up reports in a timely manner, incorrect dates and surgical procedures or death reported as the SAEs (the reasons leading to death or requiring surgical procedures are the serious adverse events).

An AE may necessitate or fulfil the criteria for subject discontinuation in a trial. Observation of certain AEs of concern in higher frequency or severity may lead to trial suspension or termination. AEs observed in a trial may have implications on other trials with that IP. The decision to stop a trial may be taken by any of the concerned stakeholders i.e. investigators, sponsor, ECs or HAs. While the sponsor may terminate the entire trial, the HAs may take the decision about their respective countries and the investigators or the ECs may take the decision about their respective trial sites.

If the new safety information is significant, it may affect the decision of trial subjects to participate or continue their participation in the trial. Hence, it needs to be informed to the trial subjects or their legal representatives. The new information is formally communicated through an amendment to the informed consent form (ICF) or a letter. Subjects could be informed verbally as an immediate measure before the amended ICF or letter is approved and available for use.

Operationally, a few decisions and activities need to be undertaken on a real-time and urgent basis such as decisions on subject discontinuation, trial termination, ICF revision or expedited reporting of SAEs. Sponsor's medical monitor may be involved in discussion with the investigators to take an appropriate decision. Data safety monitoring committee of a trial are typically involved in the decision about safety findings leading to trial suspension or termination. It is prudent to collect all necessary information from the clinical site on the relevant AEs in real time. Besides its need for immediate discussions, it is helpful for preparing narratives of significant AEs, which are usually included in the clinical study report.

Pregnancy in a female subject or female partner of a male subject while not considered AE or SAE is an important event especially when the IP has teratogenic potential and thus, has a risk to the unborn fetus. Typically, there is a provision for expedited reporting of such events to the sponsor and EC. The pregnancy is typically followed up until childbirth, and subsequently, the newborn child may be followed up for a specific duration to ascertain or rule out any malformation. The subjects may be requested for termination of pregnancy where there is a significant risk of malformation.

74. Fundamentals of pharmacovigilance operation in clinical trial

The World Health Organization (WHO) defines pharmacovigilance (PV) as the science and activities relating to the detection, evaluation, understanding, and prevention of adverse reactions to medicines or any other medicine-related problems. Prior to market authorization, a considerable amount of safety data is generated in the development process. Systematic monitoring is necessary to identify previously recognized and unrecognized safety of the investigational products (IP). The traditional focus of PV activities has been on detection and evaluation of safety signals in the post-approval environment; such methods and tools are now used in the pre-approval period.

While general clinical trial data are collected in clinical databases for individual trials, all serious adverse events (SAE) reported in association with the IP across trials in a program are entered into a safety database. It allows the PV team to monitor, assess, and report any significant safety information to authorities.

Investigators are required to report all SAEs to the sponsor within 24 hours of becoming aware of it. The PV team is responsible for receiving, seeking any clarification, analyzing, and reporting of SAEs to authorities and other investigators. The medical monitors facilitate the collaboration of the PV team with the clinical sites in this process. Email or fax is the traditional means of reporting from sites; increasingly, electronic data capture system (EDC) used for routine clinical trial data reporting is also utilized for SAE reporting. Additional fields are added to the AE page in the EDC to facilitate it. Such approach minimizes duplicate efforts and potential data discrepancies between a clinical database and drug safety database.

Traditionally, investigators are required to enter the information for SAEs both into the EDC (used by the clinical and data management group) and into SAE form (used by the PV group). Periodic reconciliation between these two databases (electronically or manually) is routine to maintain consistency.

The PV team monitors SAE notifications for individual case safety report (ICSR) processing. Typically, a multidisciplinary team led by a safety physician is responsible to conduct a primary review of individual case reports. Members of the safety team determine whether individual reports meet criteria for reporting to health authorities (HA), ethics committees (EC) and investigators. Often, PV operations are outsourced to specialized external organizations.

Databases are typically programmed to alert new entries of SAEs. All reported cases are checked for validity (i.e. presence of minimum elements - an identifiable reporter, an identifiable patient, an adverse reaction, and a suspect product) and any potential duplication (e.g. previously reported event or follow-up report). Cases are triaged based on expectedness, relatedness, and seriousness for any expedited reporting requirement with special attention to fatal or life-threatening events. The next steps are an entry into safety database, narrative writing, and medical review. Any missing or unclear information is queried to the clinical sites for clarification. It is an iterative process until the event is resolved or no further information can be obtained.

Suspected Unexpected Serious Adverse Reaction (SUSAR) refers to an SAE, which is assessed by the sponsor and/or investigator as unexpected and has a reasonable possibility of a causal relationship with the investigational product. When an SAE is judged reportable on an expedited basis, the blind is broken for that specific subject by designated personnel within the PV group for proper assessment. Events in placebo group usually don't require expedited reporting unless it is causally suspected due to an excipient in placebo. The blind is kept for other trial team members to prevent any influence on trial conduct.

SUSARs are notified to investigators, ECs and HAs in a standard format (e.g. CIOMS or Medwatch). If final description and evaluation of a case are not available within the required timeframe, an initial report is notified with the minimum necessary data followed by additional reports subsequently. SAEs in the active control are reported either to the manufacturer of the active control or to authorities.

Generally, fatal or life-threatening SUSARs need to be notified to authorities within 7 calendar days after first knowledge by the sponsor followed by a complete report within 8 additional calendar days. The report includes an assessment of the importance and implication of the finding, relevant previous experience with the same IP or similar medicinal products. The timeframe is 15 calendar days for other SUSARs.

In the context of global clinical trials, expedited reporting of SUSARs may be needed in all other participating countries as per local regulations besides where it occurred. The format and timeframe for the reporting may vary by country and requirements may change over time. Safety databases are programmed with the up-to-date regulatory reporting intelligence to automate electronic reporting of SUSARS accordingly through direct export to databases of authorities (e.g. EudraVigilance in Europe). Provisions for manual reporting to those databases are also available. Compliance with reporting is tracked and reviewed periodically.

Besides individual cases, aggregate reports along with an analysis of all safety information and assessment of benefit versus risk are submitted to the HAs at periodic intervals [e.g. DSUR (US IND-annual updates, EU annual safety updates), PSUR, PADER, and PBRER, etc].

Signal detection is an important concept in PV operation. The WHO defines safety signal as reported information on a possible causal relationship between an adverse event and a drug, the relationship being unknown or incompletely documented previously. Spontaneous adverse drug reaction (ADR) reporting systems, active surveillance systems, non-interventional studies, clinical trials, scientific literature are typical sources of information. Other relevant information such as quality, non-clinical, clinical, pharmacovigilance, and epidemiological data about IP use are also considered.

A methodological investigation is performed to assess causal relationship of a signal that takes into consideration the nature and quality of the data, strength of association, relevance, biological plausibility, consistency of the data, the exposure-response pattern, etc. This is a highly regulated process. The PV team work closely with a multi-disciplinary team of toxicologist, pharmacologist, biostatistician, epidemiologist, clinical scientist, and medical monitor to assess the safety data if there is an emergence of new safety information that changes the risk-benefit profile of the IP.

Typically, sponsor organizations have safety boards to deliberate on important safety topics relevant to investigational product safety e.g. decisions on the transition from preclinical to human phase of development, early phase to phase III of clinical development, any safety signals arising from clinical trials, preclinical experimentation, etc. Such internal safety bodies work closely with data monitoring committees (DMCs) of respective investigational products to periodically review and formulate a response to safety issues consistent with risk management plans.

Risk Management Plans (RMP) in the EU or Risk Evaluation and Mitigation Strategies (REMS) in the US are part of standard pharmacovigilance planning to minimize risks related to a medicinal product through interventions and to communicate those risks to stakeholders. Although required part of marketing authorization, it is a good practice to have it earlier during clinical development to facilitate characterization and documentation of the safety profile. It is updated throughout the lifecycle of the product and any post-authorization obligations are documented in these documents.

75. Data monitoring committee and adjudication committee

In long duration trials, the trial team directly involved in planning and execution can be biased by interim results in the trial or any significant new understanding of the disease or other therapies outside the context of the trial. It may potentially prompt them to make changes to the trial design or conduct in a way, which may compromise the credibility of the trial. However, there is a need for continuous monitoring of trial data to safeguard the health of trial subjects. Hence, an independent review of such data is essential to advise the sponsor about continuing safety of trial subjects, while upholding validity and scientific merit of the trial without jeopardizing its integrity.

Data Monitoring Committees (DMC), Data and Safety Monitoring Boards (DSMBs) or Data and Safety Monitoring Committees (DSMCs) is an independent group of experts outside the trial team who review cumulative data from one or more ongoing clinical trials on regular basis to meet such a need. It is typically recommended for controlled trials comparing rates of mortality or major morbidity. It is typically not needed in most clinical trials e.g. trials in the early phase of development or trials addressing non-critical endpoints. DMC adds administrative complexity to a trial and needs additional resources; hence, the need for DMC should be carefully assessed.

DMC may be appropriate if the trial involves following situations:

- Large, long duration, and multiple centers
- Possibility of highly favorable or unfavorable result, or futility at an interim analysis requiring early termination
- Safety concern, e.g. invasive procedure or possibility of serious toxicity with the study treatment
- Vulnerable population as children, terminally ill, diminished mental capacity or a population at elevated risk of death or other serious outcomes irrespective of the nature of endpoint

Alternatively, an entire investigational product development may be under the supervision of a DMC.

DMCs are composed of clinicians with expertise in relevant clinical specialties and a biostatistician. Experts in other fields such as medical ethics, toxicology, epidemiology and clinical pharmacology may be considered in specific situations. Representation of gender, regions, countries, and ethnic groups may be relevant, especially in international trials. Potential conflicts of interest such as financial interests or strong scientific views are important considerations. Independence of a DMC is critically essential, and members should not have any role in design or conduct of the trial. Prior experience is particularly important for the DMC chair.

The operation of DMC is governed by a charter that includes membership and other relevant issues such as responsibility of DMC chair and members, responsibility of sponsor, assessment of conflict of interest, confidentiality, schedule and format of meetings, modality of data presentation, documentation of DMC reports, record retention and procedure to amend DMC charter.

Besides occasional face-to-face meetings, it is usual to have telephonic meetings at periodic intervals.

Generally, a mechanism is established for DMC to have access to unblinded interim data and the results of comparative interim analyses to ensure DMC to identify and address emerging safety concerns. Confidentiality of the interim data is protected through agreements between sponsor and DMC members. It is essential to define modalities to safeguard such data from the trial team, investigators, or anyone else outside the DMC to minimize bias in the subsequent conduct of the trial.

DMC meetings typically have an open session in which non-confidential information such as recruitment status, baseline characteristics, screen failures, the rate of AEs or SAEs, and administrative data are discussed. External data such as published literature relevant to the study may be part of the open session. Comparative interim data or unblinded information is deliberated in "closed" sessions attended only by the DMC members. Following the closed session, the DMC typically meet with the sponsor representative(s) to convey the DMC recommendation.

The DMC recommends to the sponsor about the continuation of the trial i.e. if it could continue as planned, and typically, that is the usual outcome. Other recommendations could be trial termination, continuation with modification or temporary suspension of enrolment and/or study treatment pending further review. Minutes of each DMC meeting is documented in a brief report with the recommendation and the rationale. Any decision other than the continuation of the trial as planned may suggest unexpected events or concerns with a necessity to communicate such information to health authorities, investigators, and ethics committees. Fundamentally, it is the prerogative of the sponsor whether to comply with DMC recommendation, and it is not binding.

An Adjudication Committee (AC) is set up in certain trials to determine whether the endpoints meet protocol-specified criteria.

Such committees are particularly valuable when endpoints are subjective and require the application of a complex definition or when the intervention is not delivered in a blinded fashion. Treatment allocation is masked to prevent any bias. Information reviewed may include any relevant data such as clinical or laboratory data, autopsy reports, physical examination, etc.

Like DMC, a charter is developed for AC governance that describes composition, responsibility of the AC chair and members, responsibility of the sponsor, criteria for endpoint assessment, frequency and logistics of meetings, modality of coordination, data presentation format, methods to identify cases for adjudication, adjudication process, documentation and tracking of adjudicated cases and outcomes, and retention of records. Typically, AC is independent of DMC and members do not share any DMC responsibility as DMC can have access to unblinded information, while AC members remain blinded to treatment allocation.

From an operational perspective, important tasks are the selection of members with adequate qualification, the arrangement of the meetings at an appropriate frequency, coordination for timely availability of clean data as well as relevant records from sites for adjudication. The outcome of endpoint adjudication is entered into the database for analysis through a specifically designed eCRF page or as third-party data transfer.

76.Discontinuation and lost to follow-up

Subjects may discontinue participation before planned completion after trial entry. Investigators may withdraw subjects from a trial for specific reasons (e.g. adverse events, safety concerns, and significant protocol deviation). Lost to follow up are situations, when subjects don't show up for scheduled visits and repeated attempts to contact the subjects are unsuccessful.

Typically, subjects who discontinue prior to initiation of trial intervention or randomization are termed screen failures and are not counted as discontinuations. Besides safety concerns and protocol deviations, subjects are withdrawn for reasons such as pregnancy, consent withdrawal, trial suspension or termination and ethical concerns. Operationally it is imperative to clarify the reasons for trial discontinuations in the protocol. There can be reasons other than those foreseen at the time of protocol development. It is important to ascertain the reason for trial discontinuation, especially if suspected to be related to adverse events; as such, the reasons for discontinuations are collected in the CRF for analysis. A clear guidance should be available in the protocol on managing the subjects after trial discontinuation.

The setting of subject discontinuation may vary depending on the reason for discontinuation, availability of the subject for follow up visits and status of consent. When possible, end of study evaluations should be conducted to ensure health status of the subject is known, at the time of discharge from the trial. If required, additional follow up visits may be planned. In extreme cases, a subject may request not to analyze his or her samples or withhold data from the analysis; such situations should be managed depending on local regulations.

When a subject is lost to follow up, attempts to contact the subject are documented in the subject file. Increasingly lost to follow up is viewed with suspicion. There are concerns if subjects considered lost to follow had any serious adverse events. Sites should not hastily term subjects as lost to follow up and a reasonable attempt should be made to establish contact with the subject. The circumstances should appear plausible to a third party. Alternatively, subjects may be considered provisionally lost to follow up after reasonable efforts while a final attempt is made at the time of study completion.

When patients are withdrawn from study treatments, they may be provided with the option to receive either the standard of care or their previous treatment before entering the trial. Subjects, who have AEs and need treatment, are provided medical care as per the protocol or the standard of care to treat AE. Referral to other physicians or facilities for treatment could be considered. Generally, treatment cost is borne by the sponsor for trial-related AEs.

In the event of withdrawal, compensation to subjects for the duration of trial participation is typically prorated; however, full compensation may be considered when subjects are withdrawn due to safety reasons; local practice may vary, and it should be considered. The details of compensation for trial related injury, death, treatment cost of AE and compensation for trial participation should be explicitly described in the informed consent form (ICF), approved by the ethics committee (EC) and discussed with the subjects before enrolment. For discontinuations, investigator's fees may also be linked to the duration of subject participation in the trial.

A reasonable number of discontinuations are usually taken into consideration in sample size calculation based on the trial setting and prior experience. Once this limit is breached, the trial may lose the desired power to estimate an endpoint within reasonable assumptions. Thus, the discontinuations are closely monitored and the reasons for discontinuations are scrutinized as the trial progresses. In certain cases, the sample size might have to be increased based on the actual discontinuation rate to maintain statistical power.

Retention measures should be discussed and put in place proactively alongside enrolment. Reactive measures later are generally less effective. Discontinuations should be carefully evaluated and discussed with the site staff or monitors to understand specific problem areas. Once specific reasons are identified, appropriate steps should be attempted to address the issues including protocol amendment. There may be site-specific issues, which can be identified in a comparative analysis with other sites, in a multicenter trial.

Compliance with the protocol may be improved by proper subject selection, practical visit schedule, relaxation of study restrictions as well as regular counselling and follow up. Some of the reasons for subject discontinuations may be related to study design with little scope for improvement. If the discontinuations are due to safety reasons (e.g. increased incidence of adverse events), it may have a significant implication on the trial conduct. In extreme situations, the trial may have to be suspended to carry out a safety review or terminated.

77.Basics of monitor and monitoring

Monitoring is the process of overseeing the progress of a clinical trial, and of ensuring that it is conducted, recorded, and reported in accordance with the protocol, standard operating procedures (SOPs), good clinical practice (GCP), and applicable regulatory requirements. Operationally, a monitor is the interface between the clinical site and the sponsor as most communications between the sponsor and the clinical sites are channelled through the monitors.

As per GCP obligations and sponsor's contract with the clinical site, the monitor is authorized to have access to the relevant facilities and documents at the trial site as well as to seek clarifications on trial conduct. Well planned, adequate, and timely monitoring ensures credibility in trial conduct and the data generated in the trial. The responsibility of the monitor is not only to verify compliance but also to facilitate trial conduct as per requirements and sponsor's expectations.

The monitor is sponsor's authorized representative from sponsor's organization or another organization to which monitoring service has been delegated. Considering the crucial role and regulatory significance, monitors should be carefully selected and adequately trained commensurate with the complexity of the trial. Familiarity with the protocol, informed consent form (ICF), investigational product (IP), sponsor's SOPs, GCP and applicable regulations is essential for effective monitoring.

Broadly, monitoring covers the following responsibilities as per ICH GCP:

- Proactively maintain line of communication between sponsor and investigator
- Verification of qualification, resource, and infrastructure of the investigator and the site
- Overseeing and verification of IP handling at the site
- Verification of compliance with protocol, agreement with sponsor and regulatory requirements
- Verification of informed consent process and signed ICFs
- Ensuring availability of current trial documents and all supplies at the site
- Ensuring adequate training of the site staff
- Subject eligibility verification
- Reporting of study progress
- Checking source documents for completeness, accuracy and up to date entry
- Ensure proper documentation at site
- Verification of accurate, complete and timely case report form (CRF) entry as per the source documents, CRF entry guidelines and training, protocol or other study documents and regulatory requirements
- Verification of adverse event reporting to all concerned parties as per requirements
- Check for essential document maintenance at the site
- Informing investigator about any deviations from protocol, SOPs, GCP, agreements with sponsor and regulatory requirements as well as taking steps for its prevention

Operationally, the extent of monitoring requirement is evaluated along with protocol development. It depends on the objective, trial design, complexity, trial endpoints, assessments, and experience of the sites. Certain activities need to be entirely monitored such as verification of IP handling, whereas, others may be monitored to a limited extent such as source data verification. When limited monitoring is planned, a random sample of subjects or visits may be selected. The extent of monitoring can be revised depending on the evolving situation at the site.

It is a common practice to outsource monitoring services. The extent of monitoring work hours in terms of the number of site visits, travelling, onsite monitoring, training, project management, report preparation and other trial activities is estimated for resource management and is essential for outsourcing. The protocol and the monitoring plan are the basis to estimate the resource requirement for monitoring (manpower and cost).

In blinded trials, there may be a requirement for an unblinded monitor (who has treatment allocation information) to monitor processes of randomization, treatment allocation and drug preparation at the clinical site. The unblinded monitor is not involved in any other monitoring activities to prevent bias. Another monitor who remains blinded to treatment allocation is responsible for other monitoring activities. Any such requirements should be explicitly identified for resource planning. A communication plan needs to be established between the blinded and unblinded monitors and other personnel in the trial who may or may not be blinded to ensure unblinded information is protected.

Typically, the monitors are taken onboard during the trial planning and play an important role in site identification and selection. The monitoring group may be involved a bit later if the site management is handled by another group or only sites with prior experience with the sponsor are under consideration.

In the recent years, the approach to monitoring has been transformed to maximize the effectiveness of the overall efforts with a greater emphasis on risk-based and adaptive methods. The advent of new technologies and changes in regulatory guidance on this topic has led to a more comprehensive approach. The different approaches to monitoring have been covered in another section of this book.

Monitoring is conducted as per the protocol, sponsor's SOPs, applicable regulatory guidelines, GCP, ethics committee requirements and sponsor's agreement with the investigator. Generally, monitoring has a considerable component of onsite activity and it is not allowed to carry original site documents for review outside the site. Due to the frequent onsite travelling requirement, monitors from nearby locations are often selected. Frequently, there are backup monitors to cover absences of the regular monitors. The backup monitors should be trained appropriately.

Many clinical research professionals begin their professional careers as monitors in clinical operations domain. The structure of the monitoring team, its interface with project managers and the trial scientific team is crucial for smooth trial conduct. In large global trials with many sites, there can a reasonably big team with country or regional level reporting structure. Due to entry-level nature of the positions, a bit of churn is routine; hence, there is a constant need to train new personnel. The training should cover key aspects of the trial in a simple and straightforward manner. Monitors are generally trained to follow simple instructions and bring any issues to project managers for resolution.

Experience of the monitors with clinical sites or similar trials is of immense value, and it should be looked for in complex trials or in case of difficult investigators. Sometimes, sites may have genuine concerns about the protocol, budget, vendor services or safety of the IP, which need to be addressed. It is not unusual to have conflicts with the site personnel when the monitor points out deficiencies. The monitors should forge a working relationship with the site staff and have a constructive attitude to the support smooth conduct of a trial. Monitors should be empowered by the sponsors to be effective.

A monitoring responsibility log identifies the responsible monitor(s) at a site, for a particular trial, at any given time. It remains at the site and should be updated, when the monitor(s) are changed, to reflect the responsibility transfer. Every visit of the monitor to the site is registered in a monitoring visit log (which remains at the site). The responsibility of the monitor ends after site closeout or as per the agreement.

78. Different approaches to monitoring

Frequent periodic visits to study sites along with 100% source data verification was the preferred approach to monitoring in industry-sponsored trials until recent past. This was partly driven by such expectations from regulatory authorities. Alternate approaches have evolved with an understanding of the limitations of the conventional approach, and a changing expectation to maximize the effectiveness of the effort. Basics of different approaches to monitoring in use are described here; a combination of different approaches is the norm in a trial.

Onsite monitoring:

The monitor periodically visits the clinical site to verify source documentation, the familiarity of the site staff on protocol, protocol compliance, data entered into eCRF, investigational medicinal product (IP) accountability and disposition, site training, investigator's oversight, investigator's file completeness, etc. Role of onsite monitoring is invaluable especially early in the trial conduct to identify and rectify any errors through swift retraining of the site. Certain monitoring activities such as verification of IP, sample storage, investigator's oversight, consent procedure, etc are only possible through onsite monitoring. Onsite monitoring is typically expensive due to travel requirements.

Centralized or remote monitoring:

Certain monitoring activities when performed centrally or remotely can reduce the need for onsite monitoring visits. Data collected through eCRF or other electronic sources could be reviewed for inconsistency or incompleteness as well as protocol deviations. Site performance metrics could be evaluated and compared between sites to understand outlier sites (i.e. screen failure, withdrawal, SAEs, protocol deviation, CRF completion, pending data management queries, etc) as well as to find specific trends or patterns. Regulatory and administrative documents could be reviewed remotely when available in electronic format. IP accountability could be performed by review of IRT reports to some extent (interactive response technology). Scanned source documents uploaded to specifically designed portals can allow remote source data verification (SDV). Central monitoring can help in identifying sites for targeted monitoring.

Targeted monitoring:

In this approach, monitoring activities are focussed on specifically identified sites, key study procedures, key study visits as well as source data verification of key data elements collected in eCRF. The sites, subjects or procedures could be selected randomly or driven by predefined risk or importance. Statistical methods could be used to target a certain percentage of data elements/procedures for monitoring.

Adaptive and risk-based monitoring:

This is a relatively new concept of focussed monitoring approach to prevent or mitigate important and likely sources of error in conduct and reporting of clinical trials. Risk-based approach is applied to both processes and sites. Risks related to critical processes or data elements in the trial are identified, and a risk categorization is made based on the likelihood of error occurrence, its impact, and a possibility to detect it.

Typically, data supporting primary and key secondary objectives as well as processes related to informed consent, eligibility, IP management, documentation, adherence to key study procedures, safety data reporting, and investigator oversight are considered critical. Risk assessment and categorization of sites is performed based on prior experience and site evaluation before trial initiation, and based on site quality metrics at periodic intervals. The extent of monitoring and other interventions are calibrated for individual sites with an approach to minimize it for non-critical processes and well-performing sites. One of the key objectives of this approach is maximizing the effectiveness of the monitoring efforts.

79. Monitoring plan, SOP, visit, and report

Monitoring is a fundamental component of clinical trial operations to ensure compliance with protocol, good clinical practice (GCP), standard operating procedures (SOP) and applicable regulations. Monitoring plan is the guiding document for the monitor with necessary information and principles to monitor a trial. The monitoring findings are reported to the sponsor in a monitoring visit report. In addition, the monitoring findings are discussed with the investigator and site staff for clarification or corrective measures.

The monitoring plan is developed once a draft protocol is available taking inputs from the trial team and it should be final before trial initiation. Due consideration is given to trial design, population, assessments, and clinical sites. If required, the monitoring plan could be amended to reflect the changing monitoring needs during trial conduct. A monitoring plan broadly covers following aspects:

- Contact details of relevant team members in the trial
- List of SOPs to be used for monitoring
- Overall monitoring visit plan (visit schedule, frequency, duration)
- Roles and responsibilities of monitor and training
- List of documents such as laboratory manuals or drug administration manuals to be referred to in the trial
- Site training plan on protocol, GCP, safety data management, laboratory procedures or any special equipment used in the trial
- Specific plan on managing different visits such as site selection, initiation, routine and closeout visits
- Specific monitoring elements or any real-time observation requirements (informed consent, drug preparation, drug administration, laboratory procedure)
- Investigational products (IP), trial materials as well as biological sample storage, disposition and accountability at the site
- Supply and re-supply of various trials materials including IP, laboratory accessories, devices, paper documents, etc
- Protocol deviation management such as identification, reporting and subsequent action plan
- Source data verification plan (data elements, timing, proportion of source data to be monitored)
- Issue management and escalation
- Communication plan
- Review of site specific documentation and Investigator's file completeness
- Tools, checklists and other monitoring aids

Depending on the nature of the trial and organizational practice, monitoring plan could be an extensive document with elaborate details or a brief document with broad outlines. In large global trials, such elaborate plans are helpful for operational simplicity to minimize reliance on the judgement of monitors. If there is provision for unblinded monitor or remote monitoring, additional monitoring plans are prepared to describe such activities. In risk-based monitoring, the monitoring plan should cover the process of risk evaluation, categorization, and subsequent monitoring adaptation.

Typically, monitoring is conducted as per sponsor's SOPs on monitoring. If the sponsor doesn't have a set of SOPs on monitoring, SOPs of the service provider may be used; however, the sponsor should review and authorize its use. Typical areas where SOPs are followed include site selection, monitoring visits (initiation, routine and close out), drug accountability, source data verification, trial documentation management, handling trial termination, managing trial misconduct, safety data management, review of trial supplies and visit report preparation. Monitors should be conversant with the SOPs and complete the training before initiating monitoring activity.

Any trial has general and some specific focus areas for monitoring. GCP compliance, IP accountability, protocol adherence and regulatory compliance are the typical general aspects for monitoring. Specific focus areas of monitoring are typically the assessments to support the primary objective of a trial. All these aspects should be explicitly identified in the monitoring plan and discussed with the monitors. The extent and data elements for source data verification (SDV) should be clearly defined in the monitoring plan. In large trials, it is acceptable and practical to perform SDV in a random proportion of subjects.

The monitoring visits are scheduled by the monitor in agreement with the investigator and site staff. The monitoring visits should be planned in such a way as to get a maximum opportunity for real-time observation of key trial procedures. The typical activities in a routine visit comprise of real-time observation of identified study procedures and retrospective audit of trial activities by review of records. At the end of a visit, the monitor discusses the observations with the investigator or site personnel and reports that to the sponsor. Any corrective measures to be taken by the site should also be discussed and documented. Significant issues should be immediately brought to the sponsor's attention, while all issues are elaborated in the monitoring visit report.

In the newer approach to monitoring, certain monitoring activities can be performed remotely by review of site documents available in electronic portals, review of reported data in eCRF and telephonic discussion with site personnel. Both onsite and remote visits are planned in a way to maximize the efficiency of monitoring efforts.

A systematic approach is essential to cover key aspects of the trial in any monitoring visit unless the visit has a specific purpose. Necessary information may be gathered to complete a structured monitoring visit report. In addition, monitors should be vigilant about ethical aspects and any scientific misconduct.

The monitoring visit report typically captures various aspects of monitoring such as site interaction, recruitment progress, informed consent form review, protocol adherence, protocol deviations, IPs, trial supplies, adequate involvement of investigator, any change at the site (personnel or infrastructure), code breaks in randomized trials, trial documentation (investigator file completeness), any open issues, resolution of issues identified in previous visits, data management (data entry into case , query resolution, SDV) and so on.

Visit reports are increasingly integrated into clinical trial management systems (CTMS) and are prepared and reviewed within electronic document management systems. CTMS and visit reports can be mutually complementary as sources of trial information. For example, protocol deviations registered into CTMS can be populated to an electronic visit report automatically. The monitoring visit reports are reviewed by project managers and archived in the trial master file. In large trials with many sites, review of visit reports may be delegated to other organizations while random samples of reports are reviewed by the sponsor. A similar process of report preparation and review is also followed for remote monitoring.

80. Protocol deviation (PD)

A protocol deviation (PD) is any change, divergence, or departure from a trial protocol. Even after meticulous planning, there are chances of deviations due to several factors. PDs may be planned by the investigators for safety or logistics reasons, thus, can be immediately identified; more often, it is discovered in the retrospective review. PDs can potentially affect several fundamental principles of trial conduct and outcome.

A protocol deviation is classified as 'minor' if it is perceived not to have a significant impact on subject's rights, safety, well-being as well as the completeness, accuracy, and reliability of the data.

Examples of minor PDs

- Vital signs measured outside the protocol specified time window
- Vital signs (heart rate and blood pressure) measured in sitting position while it should have been in supine position
- Blood pressure measured in the wrong arm
- Study drug taken outside the protocol specified time in a long-term efficacy trial

A protocol deviation is classified as 'major' or as 'protocol violation' if it is perceived to affect the subject's rights, safety, or wellbeing and/ or the completeness, accuracy, and reliability of the data. A protocol deviation, which is considered as minor in one occasion, may be considered major in a different occasion. Thus, it needs to be evaluated on a case by case basis.

Example of major protocol deviations or violations

- Subject did not fulfil the entry criteria but was enrolled in the trial
- Subject continued in the trial despite meeting withdrawal criteria
- Trial subject received wrong medication
- The informed consent was not properly obtained
- Falsifying research data or medical records

Potential PDs can be foreseen at the time of protocol development and appropriate measures could be taken to minimize it. A PD management plan describes the process of identification, review, categorization, and subsequent actions on PDs. Operationally, a list of potential PDs is prepared by the trial team with a specific plan for each of the PDs. Typically, the PD list is a live document and is periodically updated as new PDs are observed with the progress of the trial or if any changes are made to the process of identification, review or categorization. A final PD list must be available before data base lock.

Apart from different categorization (e.g. GCP or Non-GCP; major or minor) for review and oversight purposes, PDs are assigned specific predefined codes to facilitate statistical analysis. For example, all PDs reported from individual subjects related to a concomitant medication could have one code. The codes are linked to action plan on the subject management or analysis such as inclusion in analysis, exclusion from analysis, discontinuation of a subject from the trial, etc.

The PDs can be identified by the (i) investigator or staff at the site (ii) monitor at the time of monitoring (iii) site personnel at the time of data entry in the electronic case report form (eCRF) (iv) data manager or the trial team during data review (v) data manager while managing discrepancies. A process should be established for identification, reporting and tracking of PDs as well as taking decisions on it. Not all PDs can be identified through database programming or retrospective review of data e.g. good clinical practice (GCP) issues. Monitors play an important role to identify such PDs.

Conventionally, PDs are documented in a PD notification form (electronic or paper) which captures information on the person reporting, time of reporting, trial and site identification, subject number, visit and time when the PD occurred, details of the PD, classification (if any), major or minor categorization, actions taken, status (i.e. open, closed or non-resolvable) and if EC notification required. Those PDs, which are considered major or significant and need to be reported in the clinical study report must be logged into or imported to the trial database for analysis.

This process has undergone considerable transformation with the widespread use of electronic data capture for data management and integration of various processes and databases. Different organizations may have some variations in the process depending on the available technical capability and trial size.

Increasingly, PDs are logged in electronically to trial systems such as clinical trial management systems (CTMS) or eCRF by personnel who may come across PDs e.g. monitors, data managers, medical monitors or authorized site personnel. Databases can be programmed to send email alerts for review and necessary action once a PD is entered. Electronic format along with web interface facilitates subsequent review, tracking, site performance assessment, pre-population in other reports (e.g. monitoring visit report) or importation to clinical databases for analysis.

The PDs are reviewed periodically by the trial team with a frequency determined by size of the trial, nature of PDs and its impact, and stage of the trial. A more frequent review during the recruitment and early period of trial is helpful to identify issues to take preventive and corrective measures. However, there should be a process for immediate escalation and management plan for major PDs as the periodic review cycle may be too late. PDs are evaluated from the following perspectives:

- Managing the subject e.g. subject meeting discontinuation criteria due to PD
- Handling of the subject data
- Requirement of database entry if all PDs are not entered into the clinical database
- Notification requirement to ethics committee (EC)
- Any intervention needed to prevent further PDs
- Trends and patterns by type, over time or across countries/sites

Minor PDs typically occur due to inadvertent logistic reasons during trial conduct at the site. Subjects generally continue to participate in the trial and the data obtained are used for analysis. In case of major PDs, the subjects may have to discontinue, the data obtained may have to be excluded from analysis or both. Impact of any type of PD is evaluated on a case by case basis by the trial team.

Subject withdrawal due to PDs may be considered when there are safety and ethical concern, or it is perceived that no meaningful data would be obtained by continued participation. The decision is taken by the investigator and the sponsor may be consulted as deemed necessary. An end of study evaluation of the subject should be performed before discharge. In trials with long-term follow up for safety after treatment (e.g. vaccine trials), subjects are generally allowed to continue unless there is an ethical concern.

The decision on data handling for analysis is taken before the database lock. There is a degree of subjective judgement in classifying PDs as major or minor. Nevertheless, classification of the PDs helps to manage it operationally in terms of directing efforts on issues, which has a greater impact. For instance, in a phase III trial, there may be thousands of PDs reported, but not all impact the trial equally. For oversight purposes, it is desirable to set the expectation on an acceptable level of different types of PDs at the beginning of the trial.

Generally, the site personnel and the monitors are instructed to report all PDs that have occurred, and the trial team takes the decision on data handling for analysis. For major PDs, all or certain data points may be excluded from analysis depending on the nature of PDs and its perceived impact on the research objective. Major PDs are taken into consideration in determining per protocol set for analysis set determination. As such, intention to treat analysis includes all subjects and data points into analysis irrespective of PDs. A sensitivity analysis may be considered to understand the impact (i.e. different analysis including and excluding the data).

Many PDs are amenable to identification by validation programming of the database. When data is entered in the eCRF, the system flags abnormal values, so that, site staff, monitor, and data manager are warned of potential PDs. In the data cleaning process, the site is queried about the accuracy of the data that looks abnormal. The trial team reviews the data on an ongoing basis and can identify certain PDs. In those situations, PD notification forms can be raised by the trial team for database entry. The database can also be specifically programmed to identify PDs with the logic taken from the protocol.

Frequent and repeated PDs may indicate training needs, capability issues or need for protocol amendment. Appropriate steps must be taken to understand the reason for the PDs and prevent its recurrence. The monitor should discuss the PDs with the investigator and ensure that corrective or preventive measures are taken. Repeated major deviations may have serious implications on trial conduct. Suspension or termination of the site may be considered in extreme situations if deviations continue despite all efforts and there is ethical or safety concern.

Sometimes, there is a tricky situation when investigators ask sponsors if certain PDs are acceptable. Sponsors or its representatives have no authority to allow PDs prospectively as the protocol is a regulatory document and is approved by authorities and ECs. However, if a deviation is necessary to safeguard the health of subjects, it is acceptable, and investigators can exercise it without the need for sponsor's approval.

Typically, PDs are required to be reported to the EC or health authority at periodic intervals or as required by local regulations. The PD notification forms or the PD listings (generated from the database) may be used for this purpose. The EC may intervene in case of a higher trend of major deviations and suggest specific measures including termination of the trial at a site. Important PDs (typically the ones perceived to affect primary or key secondary objectives) are discussed in the clinical study report and a listing on significant PDs is included in the report appendix. The original signed PD notification forms or copies are archived in the trial master file.

81.Note to file or memo

'Note to file' or 'Memo' is a document to record an unusual incident during a trial conduct. It could be related to a planned deviation from protocol, a certain decision taken, an instruction from the sponsor, an error discovered, a corrective measure taken, or clarification to a study procedure. ICH GCP (good clinical practice) guidance states that 'all clinical trial information should be recorded, handled and stored in a way that allows its accurate reporting, interpretation, and verification.' A 'note to file' or 'memo' is typically created to capture instances, which would not be otherwise documented in the existing documents.

It helps to reconstruct, clarify, and explain the context of the instance for future reference and understanding. There are controversies on the utility of notes or memo in clinical trials. While some believe it as a positive practice, others are doubtful of its usefulness.

Examples of circumstances where a note to file may be prepared:

- A discrepancy in different sections of the protocol discovered during the trial. A clarification was obtained from sponsor to follow the correct procedure. The discrepancy needs to be corrected in the next protocol amendment.
- A decision was taken to terminate the trial for a reason not specified in the protocol
- It is discovered that an earlier version of the informed consent form was signed by several subjects in the consent process and the subjects need to be re-consented.
- A sample processing method (duration of centrifugation increased) has changed during the trial and the study team was trained on the new procedure.
- The subject number was not appropriately configured in the database and it needs reconfiguration.

It is appropriate to generate a note to file in a situation that is applicable to many subjects or the trial in general and there is no available document that would capture this otherwise (e.g. ECG was extracted from the Holter recording 10 min after starting the resting period instead of 5 min as mentioned in the protocol). Protocol deviations for individual subjects should not be documented in a note to file. Many incidents or deviations can be captured in the subject file, comment sections of different forms, PD notification form, SOP deviation form, monitoring report and so on. Note to file or memo should not be considered as an acceptable alternative to the standard ways of documentation.

A responsible authorized person in charge of the trial or an activity (e.g. project manager, medical monitor, and investigator) typically signs off this document. The typical elements of a note to file are the trial identification code, study title, the name and details of the person generating it, details of the incident it addresses, details of file or binder where it will be placed, the personnel who would be informed about the incident (including the ethics committee chairperson if required) and space for signatures. Typically, it is archived in relevant sections of the trial master file, investigator's file or other appropriate binders where trial specific documents are placed.

Operationally, it is important to ensure that these documents are communicated to the relevant people and acknowledged. Local regulations may require such documents to be submitted to regulatory authorities or ECs. If a memo serves to change a procedure to some extent as an immediate measure, necessary amendment to the relevant documents must be made at the earliest opportunity. Generally, it is not appropriate to make any significant changes to the protocol through a memo.

The usefulness and regulatory acceptability of the note to file or memo in clinical trials is contentious. Arguments against such practice have been reinforced by examples of warnings from regulatory authorities, and the fact that a note to file only identifies the lapses or deviations in the trial conduct and such retrospective documentation of the incidents does not accomplish anything beyond mere transparency. Most regulatory authorities would like to see corrective measures on deviations, strong quality systems, and sound record-keeping practices. Hence, note to file should only be used in exceptional circumstances without any casual approach.

82.Protocol amendment

A protocol amendment is any modification to the trial protocol after it is final. The modification may be to trial procedures or information provided in the protocol. An amendment may be quite compelling or avoidable, and may or may not pose significant operational challenges. It is important to understand the necessity and implications, as it may demand a rework of trial planning and setup activities, and may affect the overall resource requirement. Generally, a formal amendment and version change are required if the protocol has been already shared externally (e.g. investigator, ethics committee or health authority).

Typical reasons for protocol amendment are (not in the sequence of common occurrence)

- Inconsistencies in different sections of protocol
- Health authority (HA) or ethics committee (EC) request
- New safety information availability leading to addition of safety measures
- Modification to entry criteria due to recruitment issues
- Modification to study restriction due to compliance issues
- Change in criteria of standard of care
- Change of information on the investigational products (IP)
- Change of study design (e.g. change in study duration, addition of a treatment arm, change in drug dose or addition of assessments)
- Addition of interim analysis
- Change in assessment procedure (e.g. change in sample processing method)
- Administrative information (e.g. sample shipment information)
- Change in sample size due to significant discontinuations or decision to allow subject replacement

Generally, an amendment that affects the safety, physical or mental integrity of trial subjects, a scientific objective of the trial, management of the trial (e.g. change of principal investigator) as well as quality or safety of trial IP would need approval by the EC and/or the concerned HA before implementation. This is called substantial amendment. The definition of a substantial amendment may vary as per local regulations. Examples of substantial amendments are a modification to entry criteria, dosing schedule or primary objective.

In some situations, an urgent measure, which is in deviation to the protocol, might have to be taken to safeguard trial subjects (e.g. new safety findings). Such measures can be implemented in the interest of subject safety and prior approval from EC or HA is not required. The protocol can be amended later to reflect the changes; EC and HA approvals can be taken subsequently. The implemented deviations can be captured as protocol deviations with justification.

Non-substantial or administrative changes may not require an approval from EC or HA prior to implementation. For instance, change in sample shipment address, change in study personnel, spelling error, correction of obvious discrepancy between the synopsis and protocol may fall into this category. Typically, such changes are not expected to affect the risk-benefit in the trial and consent of trial subjects. However, the distinction between substantial and non-substantial may be subjective and appropriate consultations with regulatory affairs colleagues (for HA) and investigators (for EC) can be helpful. Non-substantial amendments may be submitted as notifications to the EC and HA.

Sometimes, administrative changes are captured as 'file notes' and these changes are updated in the protocol at periodic intervals or at the time of a substantial amendment. If it is not clear, whether a change falls into the category of a substantial or non-substantial amendment, a conservative approach may be prudent.

While planning an amendment, impact on resources must be evaluated. Timelines, budget, IP supply, the scope of work of clinical site or service providers (monitoring, data management, or central laboratory) may need to be reworked depending on the extent of an amendment. Study-specific documents such as informed consent form (ICF), case report form (CRF), monitoring plan, statistical analysis plan, source document templates, and many other documents may need amendment.

Typically, amendments to the protocol are also reviewed and approved by internal scientific committees. When an amendment significantly affects the trial budget and timelines, upper management endorsement is essential. The contracts with external service providers need to be amended or change orders approved to reflect the changes in the scope of work. Substantial changes to timelines may affect dependant activities of stakeholders unrelated to the trial conduct (e.g. marketing application, product development, etc) and hence, timely communication to stakeholders is essential.

The protocol amendment must have the appropriate version and date control for identification. Application for EC or HA review and approval is similar to that for the original protocol. Other trial documents such as ICF, CRF, and statistical analysis plan are amended as necessary. Certain documents such as ICF must be approved by EC before use. Study personnel at all levels should be trained on the amended documents and procedures. Approvals, notifications, or acknowledgements as applicable must be available before implementing the amendment. For an amendment made in response to HA or EC request, an acknowledgement of submission of the amendment (complying with the request) may suffice, if locally acceptable.

Implementing a protocol amendment on already enrolled subjects has to be carefully considered. Subjects must be re-consented with the amended ICF prior to performing any new procedures. The need for ICF revision and re-consenting should be evaluated on a case by case basis. Subjects who don't accept the terms of the amended ICF must be withdrawn from the trial. New subjects are enrolled as per the amended version of the protocol and ICF.

While conducting global trials, protocols may need to be amended as per local requirements or HA/ EC requests. Typical suggested changes are an inclusion of additional safety assessment, modification to entry criteria or inclusion of additional standard of care. Exclusion of the particular country from trial conduct could be considered if the suggested changes are perceived to be incompatible with the overall trial. Alternatively, country-specific amendments could be considered.

Avoidable amendments, which could have been prevented (e.g. discrepancies in different sections of the protocol), are perceived as an indicator of poor quality of protocol development and organizations strive to minimize it. Several steps of review, quality check and stakeholder consultations are usually undertaken for this. Certain general strategies such as minimizing the information in the protocol, non-duplication of different sections of the protocol, following a sound protocol template and having standard texts for common study procedures may be helpful.

Protocol amendment could be very similar to original protocol development in terms of document management i.e. drafting, review, and approval irrespective of nature of the amendment. Frequent amendment to a trial protocol may be of regulatory concern, and it should be assessed from a quality assurance and regulatory acceptability perspective. There is a general preference to avoid protocol amendments.

Sometimes, protocol amendment is the only option to manage a situation such as new data or regulatory request. In some other situations, a protocol amendment could be disruptive, and strategic alternatives need to be considered e.g. additional study for new endpoints, extension study for longer follow up duration, an amendment to SAP for new analysis, additional clarifications in a procedure manual, opening new centers for recruitment challenges, etc. In other situations, protocol amendment could be an easy solution when timelines permit.

Time for an amendment could be chosen strategically to minimally impact on timelines. An amendment to increase the duration of a trial could be considered once recruitment is complete if such a need arises at a time when it is ready to be initiated. However, the willingness of the subjects to continue participation should be considered, as there could be significant withdrawals. When a protocol amendment is under consideration, both the impact and alternatives should be considered at the program level.

83.Premature termination or suspension of a trial

Clinical trials may be suspended or terminated in certain situations. One of the major reasons is to protect trial subjects from unnecessary risks based on new safety data or issues with trial conduct. In some cases, when the trial outcome has been conclusively ascertained in the interim analysis, the trial may be terminated, so that, the participating subjects get an opportunity to receive a superior treatment. It could also be due to an administrative reason if the sponsor cannot continue the trial due to financial reasons.

The decision on suspending or terminating a trial can be taken by health authority (HA), ethics committee (EC), sponsor, investigator, or data monitoring committee. The trial suspension is a temporary halt of trial activities until a further decision is taken (when data review is still ongoing), whereas trial termination is conclusive. This is different from circumstances of 'subject withdrawal', where the trial continues in spite of individual subject discontinuation.

The criteria for trial suspension or termination are stipulated in the protocol. It includes the data monitoring procedure as well as the suspension and termination criteria. Nonetheless, a trial could be terminated or suspended for other justifiable reasons and need not be limited to protocol stipulated criteria. The new data leading to such a decision may be from another trial, preclinical studies, or another molecule of the same class. Here are examples of reasons.

- One of the interventions has been conclusively proved to be beneficial at interim analysis, thus, continuing others is unethical
- Trial interventions are suspected or proved to pose unreasonable risk to trial subjects

- Significant issues in trial conduct pose unacceptable risk to trial subjects (e.g. repeated noncompliance with protocol or standard operating procedures at a site)
- Administrative issues (e.g. sponsor discontinues development of a drug, financial reasons)

Stakeholder management and communication are the key activities once such a decision is taken. Wider consultations may be required depending on the reason and anticipated implications to formulate a communication plan. Once all stakeholders (investigators, ECs, HAs as well as all other internal and external stakeholders) are notified, reactive clarifications about the reason or subsequent course of action should be anticipated. Technically, the protocol, informed consent form (ICF) and contract with service providers should have a clause with action plan in a scenario of trial termination and becomes the guiding principle for next course of activities.

The typical challenge for the investigators is to manage the trial subjects. It may be complicated due to the disease condition, type of intervention, subjects' response to interventions, and availability of other treatment options. Typically, there should be a plan in the protocol to manage the subjects in case of trial termination. For example, a subject may have responded very well to the investigational treatment, which was found to be inferior in the interim analysis. Consultation with the investigator, local EC and HA may be required.

One of the foremost considerations is the availability of the trial intervention found to be most beneficial. This requires consideration from an ethical, legal, and regulatory perspective. The willingness of the sponsor to supply investigational medications may not be the only consideration. It may take multiple years for a product registration and commercial availability. Subjects could be offered the investigational medications found most beneficial or taken out of the trial interventions and managed as per the standard of care. Subjects may have to be followed up for an additional duration to assess long-term safety or efficacy. Trial subjects should be approached to discuss the trial termination, plan to safeguard their health, alternatives available, as well as the schedule for an end of study evaluation.

As the literary meaning suggests, suspension of a trial is temporary. Generally, suspension of a trial refers to enrolment, but it could be to treatment, the transition to a next part of the trial and so on. The temporary halt allows time for corrective actions, review of data, protocol amendment, etc. For instance, a trial can be suspended at a site due to correctable GCP non-compliance (improper documentation) that warrants training; enrolment can be resumed after re-training. For trial suspension, clear communication about any actions to be completed before a further decision about the suspension is taken and its likely timeframe are crucial from a planning perspective.

Trial suspension or termination may be limited to one or few trial sites (e.g. trial misconduct has been discovered at a site). For instance, an EC may instruct to terminate a trial at a particular site due to adverse events. However, the ECs at other sites may still allow the trial to continue (e.g. inadequate facility to manage adverse events).

Once the phase of communication and clarification settles down, the operational process of trial closeout should swiftly progress. Regular trial activities such as monitoring, data management, study documentation, trial supply, or biological sample management would be typically continued as usual with some adjustments. Financial issues should be managed as per the contracts or standard business practice.

84.Interim analysis (IA)

An interim analysis (IA), as the name suggests is an analysis of trial data at any time prior to study completion (i.e. all subjects completing the last scheduled visit). Typically, the analysis would include available trial data at the time of IA or as determined otherwise (e.g. first IA with data until 6 months for each subject). It may be planned or unplanned and there may be one or more such analysis during the course of a trial. The usual objective is to understand safety or efficacy at specific time points and further course of the trial may depend on this analysis.

For planned IA, the specific details are stipulated in the protocol such as the time of analysis, subjects and assessment period to be included in the analysis, relevant data, any specific predefined design adjustment based on analysis or any criteria for trial termination. Unplanned IA may be conducted in response to unforeseen circumstances such as safety findings with the compound or request from health authorities and data safety monitoring board.

Data requirements for IA should be identified and activities planned accordingly. The subjects and the data elements for IA are communicated to the stakeholders. The trial sites, monitors, data management group, and central laboratories should plan their activities for IA. Typical activities are the scheduled visit completion for a required number of subjects, case report form (CRF) entry of subject data, source data verification (SDV), data cleanup, transfer of all other data from various laboratories to the database as well as finalization of statistical analysis plan. An interim database lock is required, and all activities must be completed prior to it.

The number of IA may have an impact on the power of the study from a statistical standpoint, especially in confirmatory trials. Planned IA is taken into consideration in the initial sample size estimation. When an unplanned IA is conducted, need for any sample size revision should be evaluated by the statistics team.

The loss of power due to an unplanned interim analysis could be handled by increasing the sample size or adjustment of statistical assumptions.

In blinded trials, the randomization code is made available to perform the statistical analysis. To maintain blinding, a due process needs to be followed to access unblinded IA data and results. The study design may be such that subsequent blinding is not necessary. However, necessary adjustments are required if blind needs to be maintained.

Common approaches are group level unblinding, access of subject-level unblinded data to a predefined group of people (e.g. safety board) who are independent to the trial, limiting subject level unblinded data to a certain trial personnel but limiting their role in trial conduct, or arrangements of separate blinded and unblinded teams. It is a common practice to redact subject level unblinded data in IA reports if the study would continue in a blinded manner after IA.

IA results may determine the next course of the trial. A futility assessment may be part of the IA, and the trial is terminated if futility criteria are met. Certain key data could be obtained from the interim analysis for strategic consideration of other trials. In an adaptive trial, design adjustments are predefined to be undertaken based on IA. As such, protocol amendment could be considered for any necessary modifications to the trial design. Stakeholders should be sensitized about the possible impact of the IA on the course of a trial.

85. Data management

Data management deals with various activities that enable collection and integration of clinical trial data to ensure those are of high quality, reliable and statistically sound. Data in clinical trials could be generated at various sources depending on the objective of the trial (e.g. clinical sites, laboratories, IRT, diary cards, etc). Clinical trial data must conform to CDISC standards, which determine the structure of the data that is vendor-independent and system neutral.

While clinical data management generally refers to subject data from clinical sites, separate data management functions exist to deal with other sources of data (e.g. central lab data). Often the different data management teams have to work closely to transfer data to the clinical database.

Here are broad responsibilities of the data management team in clinical trials:

- Creation of data standards and design of collection tools (CRF, diary cards)
- Database programming
- Development of guidance documents for data collection
- Development of data validation plan for data accuracy and consistency
- Development of specification for transfer of data from external sources (e.g. labs)
- Data review and discrepancy management
- Reconciliation of various sources of data with the clinical database
- Medical coding
- Metrics and tracking of various activities

A data management plan may be developed to describe the overall processes planned for a trial. Sub-specialities have evolved within data management to focus on overall management, database programming, data review and discrepancy management, and coding. In blinded trials, it may be necessary to have a separate team to deal with unblinded data. The data capture systems and databases should have such provisions and access control.

The bulk of the clinical data comes from clinical sites through the CRF. Data collection tools and other associated processes as described above are developed along with the protocol. The tools may be paper-based or electronic in nature.

The conventional approach is paper CRF, which may be time-consuming and cumbersome. The data entry personnel at the site enter the data as per CRF completion guideline. It is physically shipped to the data management team, and another set of data entry personnel enter the data into electronic databases. Various methods are used to prevent error in transcription from CRFs to databases such as use of validation checks, double data entry (two people entering the same data) and additional quality control through structured random checks.

Advantages of a paper-based system are simplicity, non-requirement of computer or internet connection at a site and lesser cost. Disadvantages are potentially poor legibility, lack of remote access, manual errors, the possibility of data loss due to selective data entry at the site, need for physical transportation, a requirement of two levels of data entry and potentially cumbersome query resolution process. Evidently, it can be time-consuming as well.

The advantages of electronic CRF systems are rapidity, legibility, remote access or review facility and the logistical convenience. The data transfer is immediate over the internet. The web-based application can be accessed over the internet; in case of laptop-loaded systems, only internet connection is required for data transfer. The electronic systems are password protected and only nominated users with necessary credentials can access it. Downsides are a requirement of computer systems and internet at the site. Errors in the electronic system can be sometimes troublesome. There may be initial issues of familiarity of the site personnel to electronic systems. Secured internet connections are preferred for access and data transmission. Increasingly, electronic systems are the norm.

Database programming is a key step in data management and it is usually initiated once a final protocol is available and an outline of data collection is final (i.e. CRF). Besides the data entry fields, the validation checks are programmed into the database for identification of discrepancies. A CRF completion guideline describes the instructions for the sites on access to electronic systems, navigation in the system, data entry, and query management. Similar plans need to be also developed for any other data collection tools.

A data validation manual describes the processes and review steps to ensure consistency, integrity, and validity of trial data. Manual reviews are essential for data elements where edit checks are not possible. It is important to identify elements to be reviewed, responsible personnel, and periodic frequency. Any specific reviews to be performed prior to database lock need to be also identified. Various programmed listings may be generated to facilitate such reviews.

Trial data in the clinical database is reviewed by the monitor, data manager, medical monitors, or other trial team members and may have a different level of access to the system. Record of any modification, the reason for such modification and identity of personnel making the changes is essential. This is a regulatory requirement to prevent any fraud or misconduct and to ensure data integrity. An audit trail is a record or track of any data entry and subsequent changes.

Clinical sites are queried for any inconsistent or potentially implausible data based on the protocol, other trial documents, or scientific expectations. Query resolution process is integrated into the electronic system in case of eCRF. For paper CRF, queries are raised and answered in paper documents (e.g. data query forms) or emails and data modification in the database is done by the data manager referring to these documents. In principle, only the investigator or designated representative can make changes to the data or authorize such changes. In case of eCRF, if the eCRF system is no more functional after database lock, query resolution can be handled as discussed in the context of paper CRF. These paper documents or emails are archived as proof like that for paper CRFs.

Data entry is the initial step of data management at the site level. Source data verification (SDV) by the monitor is the next step. It is followed by data transmission, review, and query resolution. Generally, a timeframe is decided for data entry after data generation as well as response to queries (e.g. 3 to 5 days). Similar is the case for transfer of paper CRFs to the data management team. Regular progress in data management enables readiness for timely interim or full analysis.

There could be several data sources in a clinical trial that are not managed through the CRF (e.g. data from central laboratories, IRT, imaging data, electronic diary and SAE data, etc.). Trial data in other databases are transferred to trial database electronically in a process called data transfer. Data transfer specifications are developed based on the type of data and statistical analysis requirement. Alternatively, data could be transferred by specifically designed systems that require minimal customization. The trial databases are also designed and programmed to receive such external data. Typically, test runs are performed before the actual data transfer.

Many times, developing the data transfer specification is a cumbersome process due to the complexity of data, protocol requirement, and involvement of several people. The data managers and the statisticians typically lead this activity. Generally, such data transfers are planned periodically or one time at the end of the trial.

Some of the data elements could be common between these different databases with the clinical database e.g. date of sample collection, date of randomization, adverse events, etc. For the common data elements, the data in the clinical database is usually used for analysis. Hence, periodic reconciliation between the different databases with the clinical database is an essential data management activity.

Data from clinical database and all other external databases need to be processed and specifically configured for statistical analysis. Analysis datasets are created and posted in Secure File Transfer Server (FTP) setup separately for each database. All datasets are merged before final transfer for statistical analysis and reporting. This step is usually performed after database lock.

Modifications to data management activities to allow additional data collection, validation programming, or data review are common. In large and long-term trials, complexities of the data may not be fully apparent at the trial planning stage. This may or may not be driven by a protocol amendment.

86.Data cleaning

A voluminous amount of data is generated in clinical trials at the clinical sites and laboratories, and is transmitted to trial databases. The amount of data generated depends on the scale, duration, objective, and complexity of the trial. Errors are unavoidable in recording or reporting of such large-scale data irrespective of efforts to simplify the process or adequate training. Data cleaning is a process wherein data goes through a planned process of check and review and is declared accurate by the investigators or laboratories transmitting it. Data cleaning is an integral part of clinical data management and is applicable to all types of data (e.g. clinical data, laboratory data).

The following are essential elements of data cleaning:

- Quality control procedures at the investigator site or laboratories
- Monitoring by the field monitor
- Source data verification by the field monitor
- Validation programming of database by the data management team
- Reconciliation of data in clinical database with other sources of data
- Review by the data management team
- Data review by the clinical trial team
- Confirmation of accuracy of the data by the investigators or laboratories

Here are examples of data issues that may be addressed in data cleaning:

- Inadvertent errors (reporting an extra digit for a laboratory data (e.g. 122 instead of 12)
- Missing data (all required data not collected in a visit)
- Inconsistent data (mismatch in date of SAE in clinical and safety databases)
- Non-compliance to instructions (reporting lab values in incorrect units)
- Incomprehensible data (reporting a disease diagnosis in local terminology)
- Fraudulent data (data which looks too good to be true)
- Non-reporting of adverse events (an abnormal assessment not reported as AE)
- Non-reporting of protocol deviations

Such errors are common and should be anticipated. It is a good practice to sensitize site personnel about common data reporting quality issues, edits check in the systems, and different reviews planned. Some of these could be described part of the eCRF completion guidelines. Field monitors (FM) are well positioned to discuss with sites the common errors to improve quality of data entry and prevent unnecessary data review cycles.

Typically, clinical sites and the laboratories have internal quality control mechanisms to ensure the accuracy of data. Certain clinical sites (in hospital settings) may not have such processes; however, investigators are ultimately responsible for the veracity of the trial data at their sites.

The FM may be able to identify errors in routine monitoring activities. The FM verifies that the data generated at the clinical site is transcribed correctly from source documents to the case report form (CRF) in a process called source data verification (SDV). In this process, the FM checks side by side the data in source documents with the data transcribed to CRF. SDV may be performed for 100% of data or a predetermined percentage of randomly selected data. The extent of SDV depends on the criticality of the data for the trial (e.g. supporting primary or key secondary objectives). In risk-based and adaptive monitoring, the extent of SDV may be dynamically adapted during the trial.

Due to voluminous data, validation programming is essential in the database to flag incorrect data. For instance, if the protocol allows age range of the subjects to be between 18 to 60 years, any reported age outside this range may be wrong and hence, would be flagged. The validation programs are created based on logics derived from the protocol, an expected range of values as well as a relationship between different data elements (e.g. an out of range lab data should be reported as AE or a missing assessment should be reported as PD). The database is programmed to pop up a question if there is any deviation to the validation checks. The discrepancies thus created in the system can be accessed by the data management team, and can be raised as queries to the sites for clarification.

The abnormal values could be due to inadvertent errors, protocol deviations, or adverse events. If the abnormal data is indeed correct, the person entering it confirms the data or adds an explanation for clarification. For instance, an out of range laboratory data may be deemed clinically non-significant by the investigator, hence, may not be reported as an adverse event.

Certain potential errors or inconsistencies cannot be managed through validation programming due to technological limitation. In some scenarios, there could be considerable overlap between the expected ranges of a potentially erroneous value and a valid value and it may require additional assessment of the context of the data. Additionally, a significant amount of validation programming checks adds to the number of queries for the sites. As such, it is cumbersome to add new validation programming to databases as new scenarios of discrepancies are discovered.

Hence, manual reviews are indispensable in data cleaning. Generally, data management team handles manual reviews where the logics are straightforward (e.g. inconsistencies between various data such as AE and medical history, duplicate reporting of AEs or concomitant medications, incorrect reporting in deviation to eCRF completion guidelines, etc). The review of instances that may require a more scientific understanding of the context is managed by project manages, medical monitors or specifically trained clinical reviewers. Clinical data review topic has been covered separately in another section of this edition.

Trial data is reviewed on an ongoing basis by the data management and other authorized trial team members as part of a cleaning process. Periodically, listings of various data (e.g. medical history, subject eligibility, demography, concomitant medications, AEs, laboratory data, patient-reported outcomes) are extracted from the database for review. Profiles of individual subjects (i.e. all trial data of a subject organized in a sequential manner as per visit schedule and evaluations) could also be reviewed separately for plausibility. Programs to support custom listing and visualization are increasingly used for easy review, consistency check and outlier identification. In blinded trials, certain clinical or laboratory data may reveal the treatment allocation and appropriate arrangements need to be made for review e.g. independent personnel.

Once suspected errors or discrepancies are identified, the next steps involve raising queries to seek clarification, correction, confirmation, or new data entry in the database. This is typically done by the study monitor, data manager or other authorized study personnel. The investigator or authorized site personnel need to add clarifications, make corrections, or enter new data in response to the queries. The entire process of question-answer or clarification is documented as an audit trail. Generally, the person who has raised a query is responsible to close it after a satisfactory response. However, the data manager may carry out certain actions with appropriate pre-authorization. Similar steps are also taken for central laboratory data, which is transmitted through other processes.

Reconciliation of the data between different databases is performed to prevent any data inconsistencies. For instance, for a biomarker data, the sample collection information (e.g. subject number, visit number, collection status such as yes/no, time of collection) is entered in CRF at the clinical site in the clinical database, and biomarker sample availability (yes/no) and result (value) for a subject for a given visit after analysis is entered into a biomarker database. If the sample were handled by an intermediate laboratory for logistics purposes, some information (subject number, visit, time of collection, accession number, etc) would also be available in a separate sample management database. Any mismatch or inconsistencies in the common data can be verified by a cross-check between these different databases. It is typically managed programmatically by the data management team. Generally, the clinical database is considered the reference and all other databases are reconciled against it.

Data cleaning is an ongoing process and begins as soon as trial data is entered in eCRF and available in the database. Operationally, proper planning is necessary to ensure that it continues on an ongoing basis and a significant work is not left behind close to the trial end. Metrics on data entry, SDV, and query resolution are typically monitored during study conduct. Besides the number of queries, reasons for longstanding queries need to be evaluated. Sometimes, huge numbers of queries are generated by too strict validation rules, and deactivation or adjustment of such rules in the database becomes necessary. It is not unusual to have systematic errors in data entry or abnormal data involving several subjects for different reasons. Such issues are best managed through training the sites rather raising queries individually.

In large and long duration trials, typical data cleaning cycle may stretch upto 3 to 5 months including SDV, query resolution, and reconciliation steps. This timeline can be considerably shorter in small and short duration trials. The clean data may be frozen in the database periodically to prevent any inadvertent modification. Once data cleaning is over, the investigator or the laboratories must confirm the accuracy of the data before a database is locked.

87.Clinical data review

Credible data that is adequate, accurate, verifiable, and plausible are crucial to ensure subject safety in clinical trials and to secure regulatory confidence in the results or claims based on it. Some of the requirements of GCP are (i) clinical trial information should be recorded, handled, and stored in a way that allows its accurate reporting, interpretation, and verification (ii) data are generated, documented (recorded), and reported in compliance with the protocol, GCP, and the applicable regulatory requirement(s) (iii) Quality control should be applied to each stage of data handling to ensure that all data are reliable and have been processed correctly.

Typical sources of data in clinical trials are eCRF, laboratory reports, patient or physician-reported outcome reports, SAE reports, etc. Implausible or unexpected data could be due to reasons such as data entry error, ambiguity in the protocol, deviation from protocol, lack of training, scientific misconduct or unexpected effect of investigational interventions. These reasons are often important from the perspective of quality of study conduct or protection of subject safety and rights.

Clinical data review is part of the overarching broader evolving concept of clinical oversight to enhance subject protection and the quality of clinical trial data. Advances in digital data capture tools now allow ready access to clinical trial data on an ongoing basis that provides an opportunity to understand the trial conduct remotely.

In the new paradigm, the objective of clinical data review is not only to ensure data quality but also to identify systematic errors on a real-time basis, so that appropriate corrective or preventive measures could be taken faster. The traditional method of high dependency on source data verification (SDV) by field monitors is now recognized to be resource intensive and inefficient. Similarly, validation programming of clinical databases in this context remains inadequate to capture systematic trends or patterns. In the new paradigm, SVD and data validation techniques are supplemented by analytics and visualization techniques as well as scientific interpretation of data trends and patterns.

Clinical data review is a multi-functional team effort. Field monitors, remote monitors, data managers, data scientists, analytics experts, clinical reviewers or medical monitors, pharmacovigilance specialists and project managers are involved in this activity. Clinical data review process comprises of both onsite verification and remote review of the data. Effective data review requires the support of tools for data mining, visualization, and analytics.

Specific listings on trial data such as medical history, medication history, entry criteria, concomitant medications, AEs, efficacy evaluations, laboratory evaluations, and protocol deviations, etc. are generated at periodic intervals. Data mining and analytics tools are used to generate custom listings, visualizations, and metrics. Periodic analysis of trial metrics and comparison across

276

countries or sites helps to understand any concerning trends or patterns.

Data is reviewed based on the protocol, investigator's brochure, risk management plan, data capture and reporting standard, eCRF completion guidelines, data management plan, monitoring plan, clinical data review plan and statistical analysis plan. In the new paradigm, specific elements and responsibilities are identified to minimize duplication of work and enhance accountability. Here are examples of elements and responsible personnel in general and in the context of a specific situation of adverse event review.

General:

- Field monitor- SDV, timely completion of eCRFs as per eCRF completion guidelines
- Remote monitor-protocol compliance based on electronic data; identification of missing data or low complexity inconsistent data; availability of third party data such as laboratory data
- Data manager-system generated discrepancies; data reconciliation; standardization of terms based on dictionary
- Data scientist-identification of new validation rules or modification of existing ones
- Analytics expert-formulation of site performance metrics; create visualization techniques to understand the data; identification of outliers or risk factors; risk categorization of sites
- Clinical reviewer/medical monitor-scientific plausibility of clinical data; identification of inconsistent data from a scientific or medical perspective; identification of trends or patterns
- Project managers-tracking of the progress and resolution of findings or implementation of actions formulated based on findings

Specific scenario (review of adverse event data):

- Field monitor-SDV; timely reporting of SAE to ethics committee
- Remote monitor-action taken on treatments consistent with protocol; reconciliation of medical history, concomitant medication use, AE; appropriate disposition of subject in case of AE leading to discontinuation
- Data manager-Consistency of reporting between databases; discontinued subjects have no further visits reported; standardization of terms based on MedDra
- Analytics expert-Identification of sites with high protocol deviations or AE leading to discontinuation; risk categorization of sites
- Clinical reviewer/medical monitor-appropriate action taken; appropriate categorization of AE of interest; review of SAEs/SUSARs/AE of interest; AE corroborates with Laboratory parameters
- Pharmacovigilance specialist-Incidence of AEs or severity

Typically, the clinical data review process and individual responsibilities are documented in a clinical data review plan, which is a live document amenable to periodic review and update. Documentation of ongoing review, findings, and specific actions are necessary for the effectiveness of the process. It is also essential to demonstrate effective oversight to a third party such as during inspection.

Periodic cross-functional review of the findings is necessary to formulate specific action plans for issues with trends or patterns e.g. data review may suggest a procedure is not performed at few sites due to protocol misinterpretation. It may be necessary to add new aspects to the review such as the addition of new edit checks, shifting review responsibility across function or removal of certain aspects perceived to be essential initially. The clinical data review plan is then revised accordingly.

88.Medical coding

Certain trial data such as adverse event (AE), medical history, and concomitant medication (CM) are collected as free text in the case report form. Investigators may describe such information in different terminology and an investigator may describe a similar event in different terminology in separate instances. CM may be reported as a brand name or generic name. The terminologies used by investigators are called 'Verbatim' i.e. the exact words or texts that were used.

Uniformity and standardization are essential to allow statistical analysis and interpretation of trial data (e.g. categorizing AE). This is also essential to summarize data in a study report. Medical coding is a procedure in data management wherein medical terminology are expressed using standardized, validated, and universally accepted medical coding dictionaries. The classification of multiple similar verbatim terms allows quantification of similar events. It is extremely important in multi-center or multi-country clinical trials.

Here is a list of different medical coding dictionaries in use.

- MedDRA - Medical Dictionary for Regulatory Activities
- WHO-ART - World Health Organization Adverse Reactions Terminology
- COSTART - Coding Symbols for Thesaurus of Adverse Reaction Terms
- ICD9CM - International Classification of Diseases 9 Revision Clinical Modification
- WHODDE - World Health Organization Drug Dictionary Enhanced

Two of these dictionaries are commonly used for medical coding i.e. MedDRA and WHO-DDE. The Medical Dictionary for Regulatory Activities (MedDRA) Terminology is the international medical terminology developed under the auspices of the International Conference on Harmonisation (ICH) of technical requirements for registration of pharmaceuticals for human use. It is a clinically validated international medical terminology dictionary for medical events captured in clinical trials such as AEs and medical history. WHO-DDE is a similar dictionary for international classification of medicines created by the WHO programme for international drug monitoring. It is used for identifying drug names in spontaneous AE reporting in routine pharmacovigilance as well as in clinical trials.

Coding is performed by a medical coding team on the cleaned data. Medical terms can be automatically coded if it finds an exact match in the dictionary. In situations, where appropriate terminology is not available, auto coding fails, and manual coding is required. The medical coder has to find the appropriate match among the terms within the assigned dictionary and perform manual coding. Medical monitors and investigators are consulted for appropriate dictionary term use. All auto and manually coded terms are reviewed for conformity by the medical coding team. Typically, the coded data is reviewed by a medical monitor before database lock. Certain errors such as inappropriate grouping of CM (e.g. aspirin+atorvastatin and atorvastatin+aspirin presented as different groups) can be identified during the blinded data review process before database lock.

Common issues faced during medical coding are illegible verbatim, spelling error, abbreviation use, incomplete reporting of an event, combining multiple events in a verbatim, adjective use, and separate reporting of multiple signs or symptoms of a diagnosis. Many such issues can be prevented by proactive guidance to sites on sound verbatim use. For medication coding, it is necessary to have complete information (e.g. indication, dose, and route).

Organizations involved in medical coding must have valid licenses to use these dictionaries, and there should be clarity on the version of a dictionary to be used for a trial, and modality to manage version change to a dictionary. Generally, it should be specified in the protocol or data management plan.

89. Database lock

All clinical trial data are eventually fed into electronic database systems of the sponsor or service providers. Database lock (DBL) marks the formal end of data management so that statistical analysis and reporting can be initiated. Once the database is locked, the data fields are frozen, and no data modification can take place. In blinded trials, the randomization or treatment allocation information is made available only after DBL.

All data management activities such as source data verification, data review, query resolution, data transfer from external databases, reconciliation with clinical database and medical coding must be completed in preparation for database lock. The statistical analysis plan including the statistical programmes for generating tables, listings and figures (TLFs) with the data must be final before the DBL.

The key component of DBL is the removal of edit rights from the site and data management personnel. There are two types of DBL i.e. 'soft lock' and 'hard lock'. In the former, the edit rights are only retained for the lead data manager. The soft lock allows certain quality checks to be performed by quality assurance groups before the final or hard lock when the database is considered final.

Quality assurance checks generally involve a random sample of data after soft lock but before the final lock. A certain targeted data review may be planned by the trial scientific team on the data supporting key trial objectives at this point. Soft lock also provides an opportunity to test the statistical programmes for TLFs and review of such outputs (dummy TLFs) by the scientific team. Outputs at this stage are generated using dummy treatment allocation codes and with necessary masking techniques.

There could be several databases for various trial data such as clinical, pharmacokinetics and biomarker databases; each such database is locked separately. The clinical database is linked to the data collected from clinical sites via case report form. Operationally, data analysis is initiated only after the clinical database is locked even if other data (e.g. pharmacokinetics data) is available earlier and the corresponding database is locked. This is to prevent any influence of data analysis on the clinical data.

Before final DBL, a checklist is typically completed to ensure all necessary activities are completed. A DBL memo is generated for documentation and is shared with statistics group as a go-ahead for analysis. The next set of activities are data extraction from each database, integration (including randomization codes) and analysis dataset generation before transferring to specially configured secure servers for retrieval and statistical analysis. The process remains the same for interim data analysis in the study.

Data archival is a key consideration and involves database design specifications (e.g. metadata, validation programmes), original study documents (e.g. paper CRFs, CRF completion guidelines, home diary cards), data in the raw data formats, final data files (e.g. SAS transport files, STDM files), query management logs, database lock memo as well as any logs SOP deviation. Subject data for individual sites are generally provided as read-only datasets in CD-ROM or other storage media.

It is important to understand few commonly used concepts in the context of data standards in clinical trials. The CDASH (Clinical Data Acquisition Standards Harmonization) specifies the name and type of fields that can be used for data collection to standardize the variable names in clinical databases. The SDTM (Study Data Tabulation Model) refers to standards for organizing clinical trial data after collection into clinical databases. In SDTM, the data are organized into several domains (e.g. demography, AE, conmed, lab data) in a way that each piece of data can be uniquely identified (e.g. a lab data for a subject is identified by subject number, visit number, the name of test, value, unit). ADaM (Analysis Data Model) is created from

STDM datasets and it defines the analysis datasets and standards for subject-level analysis. It provides a connection between the SDTM datasets and final statistical analyses.

Database lock is a major milestone in clinical trial operation as many activities must be coordinated with various stakeholders for completion such as monitoring, data cleaning, data review, and any assessments at third-party laboratories. Typically, a high-level summary of the result is expected in a few days from the database lock (i.e. flash results or first interpretable results). It is closely followed by formal study report preparation. Statistical programmes must be ready prior to DBL to provide the analysis in an expeditious manner. From an operational perspective, close communications with stakeholders and follow up is necessary for seamless progress preceding or following DBL.

In trials with long recruitment period, considerable activities could be completed long before DBL for a majority of subjects as the first set of enrolled subjects complete the trial earlier. It is important to minimize backlog close to DBL. All stakeholders and site personnel should be sensitized about timely completion of subject visits and associated activities for the last set of subjects in preparation for DBL. Intractable situations are not uncommon prior to DBL e.g. pending visit completion of few subjects or certain irresolvable data issues. Generally, it is acceptable to proceed with DBL without resolution of certain minor issues with appropriate documentation. For example, a few subjects not returning for scheduled visits could be considered protocol deviations, and the database could be locked without that data.

Database unlock is a process to unfreeze data fields to allow modification. It may be necessary if significant discrepancies are noted in the data subsequent to database lock. Usually, it is considered as an indicator of poor quality of work and is a key quality metrics at an organization level. The need for database unlocks to make the correction in the database should be carefully considered especially from the perspective of its impact on analysis and data interpretation.

Not all discrepancies need to be corrected in the database itself. Database unlock can be avoided for minor errors with an explicit description in the clinical study report. However, this approach could be problematic for subsequent data analysis as the errors remain in the database. For any database unlock after initial lock, the reason for unlocking, data elements modified, and its impact are documented. Typically, this is a controlled process with the need for senior management approval. Re-locking the database has a similar process as the initial lock.

90. First interpretable result or flash result

A formal full analysis and clinical study report generation are time-consuming. A First Interpretable Result (FIR) or flash result is an informal brief document summarizing the key results of a trial a few days (usually within 2 weeks) after the database lock. FIR describes a high-level summary of the trial results from analysis on primary and key secondary objectives for internal use and decision-making. Based on this report, significant outcomes on efficacy or safety can be communicated externally.

Results from key trials in the development program are eagerly awaited by various stakeholders both internally and externally. While a full report preparation is underway, the FIR provides the key results for appropriate interpretation, planning for additional analysis, assessment of the impact on the program, and development of communication plan. It is common to hold series of meetings with senior management and external key opinion leaders to present the preliminary results and deliberate on its potential implications.

Strategic decisions could be made depending on the nature of the trial and its results based on the FIR without waiting for the full report. For example, failure to achieve primary endpoint in a phase 3 trial may lead to termination of the development program along with other ongoing trials. A favorable outcome may lead to the acceleration of other trials, submission preparation, and commercial planning. Early phase trial results from dose ranging trials may decide the dose regimen for phase 3 trials, which could then be initiated. Amendments to ongoing trials may be necessary depending on the nature of trial results.

FIR as such is an informal document, and it is typically not shared with health authorities or ethics committees. However, important results may be communicated before a full CSR is available depending on the nature of the trial and its outcome. It is a good practice to share the results from the preliminary analysis with the trial investigators in important trials before a formal clinical study report is available. As such clinical study reports are signed off by investigators.

A brief communication may be sent out before such information is made public as sponsors typically make public statements for results in major therapy defining trials. In long-term trials, the results from interim analysis could be presented to investigators in a face-to-face or telephonic meeting and it is viewed positively. Time of disclosure to an investigator, the extent of disclosure, nature of blinding requirements after interim analysis, etc. need to be carefully assessed and corporate communication group involvement may be necessary.

The statistics team usually leads this deliverable and preparation starts prior to database lock. Selected statistical analyses are prioritized for FIR and the format of result presentation is worked out in advance. Once the results are available, intense deliberation on the correct interpretation is common depending on the complexity of the trial. Results may not be straightforward, and it is common to have ad-hoc analysis based on preliminary results. It is a good practice to discuss with the statistics and programming team in advance on the potential need for additional analysis.

Typically, there is minimal involvement from the operations team on the preparation of this brief report or its interpretation. However, there could be implications on the trial conduct depending on the nature of results, and hence, preparedness any adverse outcome is essential. Considerable coordination may be required with various stakeholders if any modification to the trial is contemplated. Additional information may be required from the sites, service providers, or external laboratories with short notice; hence, stakeholders should be sensitized well in advance.

91. Data analysis, interpretation and report writing

Data analysis, interpretation, and report writing are some of the final scientific activities in trial operation. Once all the clinical and laboratory data is available, and the database is locked, the process can be initiated. Data analysis is performed as per the statistical analysis plan and operationally, unless it is final, the database cannot be locked. Data interpretation and report writing are initiated once statistical outputs on data analysis are available. Nonetheless, preparations for such activities are initiated much in advance.

Statistical analysis plan (SAP) details the parameters, statistical procedures, outputs (Tables, Listings, and Figures: TLF) to be generated as well as the statistical algorithms to be used for analysis. It is prepared by the statistician and statistical programmer with inputs from the trial team. A protocol is the basis for this document and it can be initiated once a final protocol is available. SAP may be required by regulatory authorities along with the protocol for review. To keep the core SAP concise, the TLF shells (i.e. blank formats of final outputs) are prepared in a separate document.

A considerable back and forth discussion is common on the TLF shell format depending on the endpoints and complexity of the trial. Organizations generally have standard libraries for such statistical outputs, which can be customized for individual drug development programs and individual trials within a program. Many data elements and its presentation formats are typically common irrespective of the objective of the trial such as demography, medical history, medication history, concomitant medications, AEs, SAEs, subject disposition, screen failures, and protocol deviations. Certain efficacy, safety, or laboratory parameters are unique to individual programs or trials and so the presentation formats. Some degree of standardization is the norm for ease of data interpretation across studies within a development program.

Data analysis in clinical trials is sensitive from a regulatory perspective; hence, organizations generally have SOPs (standard operating procedures) to manage it. Broadly, the data outputs provide subject or group level data in different treatment arms. Listings present individual subject data in a preferred sorting order. For instance, blood pressure data may be listed in the sorting order of treatment, subject, visit, examination date, and time. Group level summary of data with descriptive statistics are presented for each treatment group side by side for comparison (e.g. mean, standard deviation, median, range, proportions, etc.). Depending on the objective, comparative analysis between different groups is performed to estimate statistical significance. Similarly, graphs (figures) are prepared on both subject and group level data. All these output formats of various parameters are determined before database lock.

If additional unplanned analysis needs to be performed after database lock and initial analysis, the SAP amendment may be required. Changes to analysis methodology of key trial objectives (e.g. change in primary analysis) are generally not allowed and are discouraged at this stage. Protocol amendment would generally be required for any significant SAP amendment as it must be in-sync with the protocol. Additional exploratory or descriptive analysis is common after an initial review of the results and formal SAP amendment is generally not necessary.

A first interpretable result (FIR) in the form of a brief report with high-level result and conclusion is available shortly after database lock and sets the tone for data interpretation and report writing. A thorough interpretation of the results and evaluation of its implications may be time-consuming. The data is looked from various angles and in different sub-groups. Additional analysis and comparison with previous data in the program or literature data are required for proper interpretation. Any unexpected results are analyzed to understand the basis of such outcome. In many occasions, the results are not straightforward or conclusive leading to intensive discussions and consultations. Certain trial results may have a serious impact on the ongoing clinical trials or product under development.

The protocol, SAP, and statistical outputs are the basis for writing the CSR. It should be in a prescribed format or template depending on the purpose. Report for internal decision-making such as FIR usually has high-level information, which would be adequate to understand if the major study objectives were met. There is clear guidance available on the content and format of CSR and it is followed. Here is an outline of CSR as per the 'ICH E3 guidelines-structure and content of clinical study report'. The broad headings listed below, and each has several sub-headings.

1. Title Page
2. Synopsis
3. Table of contents for the individual clinical study report
4. List of abbreviations and definition of terms
5. Ethics
6. Investigators and study administrative structure

7. Introduction
8. Study objectives
9. Investigational plan
10. Study patients
11. Efficacy evaluation
12. Safety evaluation
13. Discussion and overall conclusion
14. Tables, figures, and graphs referred to but not included in the text
15. Reference list
16. Appendices

Besides the core study report, many supporting documents (e.g. ethics committee details, bioanalytical reports, etc) are presented as an appendix to the study report. Considerable administrative details of the trial are included in the report (e.g. facilities, investigators, ethics committee, audits, laboratories in the trial, etc.). Operationally, it is a compilation of several documents from different sources besides the core report. Hence, the core report and all other supportive documents should be available in time for final publication. A full clinical study report for regulatory submission is an extensive document and may run into thousands of pages.

Usually, clinical study reports are the basis for the external publication of results, public disclosure of results and regulatory submission. Similar to the trial protocol, it is a multi-functional effort involving several personnel with iterative cycles of review and edition. In specialized environments, medical writers draft the report with help of the trial team. This model has been shown to bring more standardization and efficiency. Any modification or additional report from subsequent data analysis can be included as an amendment or addendum to the existing report, respectively.

Data analysis and report writing are among the last set of activities of trial operation. Hence, often it comes under timeline pressure if the upstream timelines were not met. Appropriate planning and follow up is necessary for timely report publication.

Drafting of the trial report shell begins even before the database lock. Many appendices for the trial report have no dependencies with the statistical output and it could be completed well in advance. Generally, a study report should be completed within one year from last subject last visit in trials in adult subjects and within six months of trials in pediatric subjects. Organizations may have shorter target timelines as per internal procedures to comply with above timeframes and to meet regulatory submission or public disclosure requirements.

Increasingly, study reports are prepared and published within electronic document management systems. However, there is no uniform standard, and the process may vary in different organizations. Typically, there are quality checks and layers of review to ensure accuracy, consistency, as well as regulatory compliance. Finally, the original report, any amendment, or addendum is signed by the authors and the investigators. In a situation, where the interim study report may have unblinded information, it is may be acceptable to not have the investigator's signature.

92. Invoice management

In a clinical trial setting, the total contracted expense for an outsourced service comprises of fixed cost (e.g. ethics committee fees), unit-linked cost (e.g. per subject screening cost) and incurred expense (e.g. sample shipment cost). The fixed and the unit linked cost is divided into a payment schedule linked to key trial milestones (e.g. contract execution, ethics committee approval, regulatory approval, trial initiation, first patient first visit, last patient last visit, database lock, trial close out, draft report availability, report publication), whereas the incurred expense is reimbursed in an ongoing manner. Sometimes, there may be an incentive in the form of monetary payments for quicker recruitment in clinical trials.

The terms and conditions of invoice management are included in the contract. Thus, an invoice received for payment is reviewed against the contract. The currency of payment, local or international taxes, customs duties and other government taxes are taken into consideration and it should be clarified in the contract. Typically, invoice management is under the purview of sponsor's project management, outsourcing, and accounts departments.

For a milestone-linked invoice, the trial project manager verifies the milestone as well as the fixed and milestone linked cost. For instance, if 10 subjects were screened, 5 subjects were randomized, and 4 subjects completed the trial, these numbers and milestones are taken into invoice calculation. Such invoice generation is greatly facilitated by integrated clinical trial management systems (CTMS) due to ready access to trial milestones and actual subject visit information by each site in a large-scale trial. Certain unit-linked expenses may be based on the trial duration (e.g. expenses for an equipment rental). Invoices for incurred expenses should be accompanied by supporting bills. Any discrepancy in the invoices should be clarified.

Once verified by the project manager, an invoice is processed by the accounts department for payment. Generally, funds are allocated for each executed contract, and any corresponding invoice is paid out of it. If the invoice value exceeds the allocated fund (e.g. extra service taken, cost increase due to unforeseen reason), the contract has to be amended by the outsourcing team before the invoice can be processed. Typically, management approval would also be required for substantial additional fund requirement. For flexibility of day-to-day operation, some flexibility may be allowed as per organizational policy (e.g. no management approval for expenses upto 5% above the contract value or 100, 000 USD whichever is lower).

The service providers should be advised to timely raise invoices and similarly, it should be processed and cleared swiftly as per the contract. There may be a penalty or late payment charges for a delay. Sometimes, invoice payment may be withheld, or penalties are imposed due to unsatisfactory work. As per local regulations, taxes may be deducted by the sponsor before payment; tax deduction certificates should be provided in such cases. Timely invoice payment is important to maintain a good relationship with service providers and prevent any unpleasant situations due to late payment.

A clinical trial may have several service providers and each with a different schedule of payment. All invoices should be tracked for the receipt, approval, and payment clearance. Increasingly, well-organized electronic systems are used for invoice management. Such systems are logistically advantageous with facilities for invoice review, approval, and tracking in a paperless environment. There are specialized organizations that support trial invoice payments and could be considered in large-scale trials.

Invoice management may be very complex in real life. Trial timelines often slip resulting in cost escalation. The scope of work frequently changes in the course of trial leading to budget revision. Service providers may not raise invoices in a timely manner or mix up invoices of different projects. Many times, these issues become hurdles in timely invoice payment and lead to significant wastage of time.

From accounting perspective, the trial budget allocated to a particular financial year need to be spent during that year. If the services have been availed but payments could not be released, it is considered 'outstanding liability' in accounting terminology. Often, there is difficulty in processing invoices of one financial year in the subsequent years due to standard accounting practices. All these complexities should be handled as per organizational procedures and local regulations.

93. Retention of investigational product sample

Retention samples are reserve investigational products (IP) that are stored at the clinical site for re-test purpose after the trial is over. ICH GCP states that it is the sponsor's responsibility to 'maintain sufficient quantities of the investigational product(s) used in the trials to confirm specifications, should this become necessary, and maintain records of batch sample analyses and characteristics. To the extent stability permits, samples should be retained either until the analyses of the trial data are complete or as required by the applicable regulatory requirement(s), whichever represents the longer retention period.'

One of the key requisites is that the samples should remain in the responsibility of the organization that conducted clinical part of the trial. The objective is to prevent sample substitution by the sponsor. While the principles are similar, the quantity and duration of IP sample storage requirement may vary by country. It may also vary according to the type of drug product (e.g. small molecules, biologics). Thus, the concerned regulatory guidance should be followed.

Guidance from Indian health authority (for small molecules):

- Quantity: sufficient to carry out twice all the in-vitro and in-vivo tests required during bioavailability / bioequivalence study
- Duration: a period of three years after the conduct of the study or one year after expiry of the drug, whichever is earlier

Guidance from US FDA (for small molecules):

- Quantity: enough quantify to permit FDA to perform five times all of the release tests required in the application
- Duration: 5 years

Guidance for operation from US FDA (for small molecules):

- Retention samples should be kept at the testing facility where the study is conducted
- The study sponsor should provide the testing facility with a supply of the test article and the reference standard sufficient to complete the study and retain the appropriate number of dosage units as reserve samples
- The study sponsor should not separate out the samples to be reserved prior to sending the batches to the testing facility
- The testing facility will randomly select the reserve samples from the supply sent by the sponsor
- In the event that a testing facility is unable to retain the reserve samples, a third party should be contracted to retain the samples

The IP must be stored in appropriate temperature and humidity with regular monitoring. There should be appropriate safety measures for such long-term storage in consideration of the importance of these IP samples. Operationally, it should be assessed part of trial feasibility evaluation and the procedures should be worked out with the clinical sites well in advance. Generally, retention sample management is not a problem at clinical research organizations routinely involved in bioequivalence trials. It could be an issue in trials in hospital settings. Independent storage facilities could be considered in such cases.

94. Investigational product (IP), biological sample and trial material disposal

Investigational products (IP), back up biological samples and other trial materials including equipment must be disposed appropriately at the clinical sites periodically during the trial or at the end. There are regulations governing disposal/destruction of biological or chemical substances, and only authorized organizations can carry out such activities; typically, it is outsourced to such organizations. The operational aspects may be included in the protocol or another document (e.g. procedure manual). Organizations generally have SOPs covering such activities.

Trial equipment, devices or computer systems supplied by the sponsor or other service providers should be retrieved once the trial is over or earlier as appropriate. If certain equipment would be gifted to the trial site at the end of the trial, it must comply with local regulations. It may not be permitted to leave behind expensive equipment at the clinical site due to conflicts of interest issues.

The time of IP destruction or retrieval depends on the context of trial supply, packaging, and treatment duration. It could be performed periodically in long duration trials once it is determined that certain IP will no more be used, once the last subject completes trial treatment or at the end of the trial in short-term trials with bulk medication supply. A final reconciliation of the IP should be carried out and accountability documented before destruction. In a trial using IRT, reconciliation, accountability, and identification of the IP to be destroyed or retrieved could be determined remotely to large extent. Generally, verification by a trial monitor is usually necessary.

Authorized facilities are used for IP destruction, and certificate demonstrating the destruction is obtained to file in trial master file. The sponsor may retrieve the IP to destroy, resupply to other sites, or use in other experiments. Retrieval for further use is practically cumbersome in most instances due to time for transportation, verification of stability in the entire course of transportation, relabeling, and packaging.

Duplicate aliquots (backup) of biological samples are often planned as a contingency measure for problems in sample shipment or analysis. In some cases, it is stored at the clinical site until the primary aliquots are analyzed and the outcome is satisfactory. The intention is only to retrieve the backup aliquot in case of any issues. In other situations, the backup aliquots are shipped to the analytical laboratory and further storage or destruction is managed there. The backup samples should be always shipped to the analytical laboratory in a separate shipment after the primary aliquots have reached. There could be leftover samples after the intended analysis is complete. A process similar to IP may be followed for the backup or leftover biological sample disposal. Stability of the sample and analyte is taken into consideration for the duration of storage.

Backup or leftover biological samples could be of immense value for exploratory research. In certain situations, there is a genuine need to analyze the backup samples to answer critical safety questions e.g. if a medical condition existed before trial medication administration or it occurred during the trial. There may be a need to analyze a new laboratory parameter, which was not foreseen at the time of trial planning.

As the purpose of sample collection and planned analysis are clarified in the informed consent, there are ethical constraints to such unplanned analysis. Concerned ethics committee may be consulted for approval of such analysis or fresh consents may be obtained from subjects is possible. It is a good practice to seek optional consent at the time of trial entry for potential future use of biological samples. Subjects may deny such use but still could participate in the trial. Information on such optional consents could be obtained in the eCRF to facilitate sample management after analysis.

In many occasions, equipment such as centrifuge, refrigerator or infusion pumps are made available at the clinical sites to facilitate trial conduct. The sponsor may purchase equipment for the sites or take it on rent from suppliers. Retrieving purchased equipment may be challenging at the end of the trial, as there may be space constraints at the sponsor location or the clinical sites. Local regulations may prevent gifting it to the sites for future use. These potential issues should be considered during trial setup, and the disposal plan should be worked out well in advance.

95.Site closeout

Site closeout officially marks the end of a clinical trial at a clinical site. Typically, the field monitor visits the site for a final review of all trial activities. The clinical site or investigator is formally notified about end of the trial and is reminded about continued obligations after closeout. Preparation is required at both sides (sponsor and clinical site) for a satisfactory site closeout, which is a requirement as per good clinical practice. A meticulous closeout visit ensures audit and inspection readiness at the clinical site.

Site closeout must be performed irrespective of the manner of trial completion (e.g. completion of scheduled visits for all subjects in the natural course, premature site termination by a sponsor, investigator's decision to terminate trial). Generally, if the site did not enrol (no subject has signed an informed consent) any subject, a formal site closeout may not be necessary. The situation should be evaluated on a case by case basis considering local regulations and practices. In any case, elements of site closeout such as the return of trial materials, payment of invoices, documentation requirement, and notification to ethics committee are typically needed.

Technically, the trial closeout could be conducted anytime after the last subject at the site completes the end of study evaluation. However, the most appropriate time is after completion of data management activities at the site or after database lock. It is prudent not to delay this, as there may be changes or loss of interest at the site over time due to changing priorities or staff attrition. It may also be difficult to retrieve certain records as time passes by.

The monitor prepares the site, and schedules the closeout visit similar to a routine monitoring visit in collaboration with the site. The sponsor's study manager should work with the monitor to identify activities to be reviewed, completed and any pending documents to be collected from the site. A checklist may be completed to determine site readiness for closeout. A similar checklist may be completed in the closeout visit monitoring report. Here is a broad list of activities to be reviewed or completed on or before the closeout visit:

- All routine or safety follow up visits of subjects completed

- Completion of data management activities:
    - All case report forms (CRF) shipped or data entered into eCRF
    - All outstanding queries resolved
    - All source documents or subject records appropriately completed
    - All protocol deviations reported to sponsor, evaluated by sponsor, filed in the regulatory binder and reported to ethics committee(EC) as applicable
    - CRF data provided and data accuracy memo obtained from the investigator

- Inventory of biological samples collected in the trial:
    - Shipment of biological samples to the sponsor, central laboratory or analytical laboratory
    - Destruction of backup samples or a plan for disposal of samples
    - Reconciliation of the biological sample inventory as well as documentation of appropriate storage and transport or plan for disposal

- Inventory of all investigational products (IP) and labels (completion of drug accountability):
    - Return or destruction of remaining IP or labels

- If not returned or destroyed, a plan for IP disposal
- Retention of IP samples at the site if applicable
- Archival of records of shipment, storage as per instruction, dispensing, accountability log in the trial master file (TMF) or pharmacy records as applicable
- Archival of randomization list, code breaks, and documentation of any emergency unblinding if applicable

- Inventory of other trial materials, instruments or supplies (documentation of return, destruction or other methods of disposal)

- Review of the investigator's file for completeness

- Notification to EC by the investigator about the end of trial

- Posting of any outstanding invoices to the sponsor for payment

- Financial disclosure from investigator or sub investigator as applicable

- Discussion with the site for the possibility of sponsor audit or regulatory inspection

Typically, the closeout visit is attended by the investigator, site coordinator, and other key personnel. Besides the above activities, review of lessons learned, and possible improvement areas could be discussed. This is particularly helpful if the sponsor routinely conducts trials with that site. It is also an opportunity for the monitor or the sponsor to mend any misunderstanding during the trial conduct to maintain a lasting professional relationship with the site.

Few activities may remain pending at the time of site closeouts such as IP destruction, backup sample disposal or trial materials return. Queries on trial data may come up later for clarification. The trial obligations even after the end of the trial should be discussed with the investigator. Typically, this should also be explicitly mentioned in the contract. A closeout monitoring report is prepared with details of the activities, outstanding issues, and the agreed plan of action. Finally, all involved parties should be formally informed about the site closeout.

Remote closeout visits could be performed in some situations and are acceptable alternatives to onsite visits. The meeting is organized as a telephonic review of the above-discussed activities and a checklist is completed jointly by the monitor and the investigator with signatures to document the review of necessary activities and pending action items.

96.Final archival of trial documents

Clinical trial documents are archived as per regulatory requirements, and it is a key deliverable of clinical trial operation. Clinical trial conduct is often subjected to audit and inspection by health authorities, ethics committees, or independent auditors appointed by sponsors. Proper archival of documents help to reconstruct the trial and maintain an audit trail.

Trial documents are archived in the trial master file (TMF) at sponsor's location and in the investigator's file (IF) at the clinical site. Some of these documents may be archived in electronic format in storage devices (e.g. CD-ROM) or electronic document management systems. Subject files may be archived separately as per institutional policy at the clinical site.

The process of ongoing record-keeping and documentation has been discussed in other sections. Final archival at end of a trial is discussed here. As per ICH GCP, essential documents (investigator or sponsor specific documents) should be retained until at least 2 years after the last approval of a marketing application in an ICH region and until there are no pending or contemplated marketing applications in an ICH region or at least 2 years have elapsed since the formal discontinuation of clinical development of the investigational product.

Since the time of marketing application may vary depending on the sponsor's strategy and phase of drug development at the time of a trial conduct, archival is typically made for a reasonably long-period i.e. 15-20 years. However, any requirement for a longer archival period should be taken into consideration. Usually, the archival requirements are described in the protocol and are part of site feasibility evaluation.

Operationally, most trial activities are completed at the time of the study report finalization. At this time, most documents are also available. It may be a good time for the final archival once the study report has been submitted to the local health authority and ethics committee. Increasingly, electronic TMFs are replacing paper TMFs, and it has several advantages in terms of convenience, easy accessibility, quality of documentation, risk mitigation, time and cost saving and audit friendliness. However, it is not widely in use now. Occasionally, when organizations may not have the required facility for long-term archival, third-party locations can be utilized.

Generally, the archival facilities should be built in a manner to protect the documents from water, fire, termite, and reasonable natural calamities. The facilities should also have backup procedures for document preservation in the event of accidents or natural calamities. A reasonable approach is to keep an additional set of scanned copies in electronic format at a different location.

97.Dates of study completion, end of trial, and primary completion

There is no universally accepted definition of the end of the trial and thus, it should be clearly defined in the trial protocol. Generally, end of the trial is considered when the last subject completes the last visit or the last data from the last subject has been generated. As there is a possibility of drug-related adverse events after last treatment administration, a pre-defined timeframe (e.g. 30 days) is also taken into consideration.

This milestone is particularly important as certain regulatory notification or reporting obligation is linked to this milestone. For global trials, this timeframe is decided by the last subject globally. Health authorities and ethics committees have obligation to oversee or monitor trial conduct in their jurisdiction and hence, must be notified of the end of trial as per local regulation. There may be a periodic fee for such supervision responsibility, which ceases after the notification. The definition as per local regulations needs to be understood to for any trial-related responsibilities once this milestone is reached.

Study completion date in US regulations is defined as the date the final participant was examined or received an intervention for purposes of final collection of data for the primary and secondary outcome measures and adverse events (for example, last participant's last visit), whether the clinical study concluded according to the pre-specified protocol or was terminated.

The EU directive states 'Within 90 days of the end of a clinical trial the sponsor shall notify the competent authorities of the Member State or Member States concerned and the Ethics Committee that the clinical trial has ended. If the trial has to be terminated early, this period shall be reduced to 15 days and the reasons clearly explained'. As per EU regulations, the sponsor is required to provide a summary report of the study within one year of the end of the complete trial for non-paediatric clinical trials. For pediatric trials, the report needs to be submitted within six months.

As per US regulations, the standard submission deadline in clinicaltrials.gov for results information is no later than one year after the study's 'Primary Completion Date' defined as the date on which the last participant in a clinical study was examined or received an intervention and that data for the primary outcome measure were collected.

However, many trial activities are yet to be completed at this point, and many sponsor obligations remain at this milestone. Sponsors and contract research organizations (CROs) may have an internal definition of the end of the trial to suggest no pending activity for a trial.

98. Modalities of communication with clinical sites

Effective communication with the clinical sites is crucial for the success of trial operation. It is needed in varying contexts such as protocol clarification, study update, availability of a latest version of a study document, new safety information, etc. The modes of communication are tailored to the situation. Nature of the trial, number and location of trial sites, type of information and involvement of outsourced organizations to manage trial operations are important considerations.

Typically, field monitors are the main point of contact from the sponsor side and site co-ordinators are the main point of contact from the investigator side. Emails, telephonic and face-to-face conversations are common and are not the topic of this discussion.

In the initial period of trial conduct, sites frequently require clarifications on aspects of the protocol and related procedures. Newer electronic platforms are now available to direct the protocol enquires in an efficient manner to the appropriate personnel, escalation to the relevant personnel as necessary with documentation of the responses and tracking. Such platforms could also serve as a repository of previously answered questions for future reference and review.

Clinical trial investigator portal is often used in larger trials to facilitate the exchange of information and training of site staff. It could be a study-specific setup or part of a larger platform covering multiple trials of a sponsor or contract research organization (CRO) with controlled access. Such platforms can be used by authorized personnel from the sponsor, CRO and the clinical site for exchange of documents (e.g. feasibility questionnaire, protocol, investigator's brochure, signature pages, safety reports, training materials) and information (e.g. updates on payments, enrolment, and study status). Such portals allow multi-directional information flow with facilities for tracking and reporting on information acknowledgement.

In large multicentre trials, newsletters are a common means to periodically update clinical sites on trial progress, remind key protocol procedures, sensitize upcoming milestones, or reiterate important logistic processes. It is usually of few of pages length, and the frequency could vary from once every few weeks to months depending on the stage of the trial. Typically, these are sent out by emails or posted in trial portals. A newsletter is a powerful tool to recognize the performance of individual sites in a way to encourage healthy competition. A bit of creativity is essential to draw the attention of sites on important messages in the newsletter in long-term trials.

Key focussed messages such as a delay in the trial initiation, important safety finding, or termination of the trial are usually provided to investigators directly by sponsor's medical leader or project manager. It is a good practice to have a telephonic discussion before sending out a written communication in a signed letter. Such letters are written in such a way that it can be submitted to the ethics committee for information.

99. Quality in clinical trial

Quality has been defined in ICH Q9 guidance as 'the degree to which a set of inherent properties of a product, system, or process fulfils requirements'. Clinical trials are conducted under strict regulatory and ethical framework to safeguard trial subjects as well as to ensure data integrity. Quality has been specifically emphasized in ICH GCP guidance. Organizations involved in clinical trials should have quality systems to bring credibility to the trial data and the conclusions derived from it.

A quality system is a management system to direct and control an organization with respect to quality. There are three broad objectives of such a system (i) to establish, implement and maintain a system which would be able to facilitate clinical trials conduct and data integrity in a manner that meets requirements of subject safety, health authorities and other customers (ii) to develop and implement a monitoring mechanism for quality assurance of clinical trial conduct and data integrity (iii) continued improvement through identification of quality issues and implementation of remedial measures.

The two major enablers of a quality system are knowledge management and quality risk management. Knowledge management refers to a systematic approach to acquire, analyze, store, and utilize information from all internal and external sources to manage the processes of clinical trial conduct. The latter refers to a system to proactively identify, evaluate, and control potential risk to clinical trial quality. Both of these enablers facilitate to achieve the quality objectives.

A quality system of an organization comprises of appropriate processes, resources, and responsibilities to deliver the quality of both its own businesses as well as its outsourced activities. In relation to clinical trials, while some of the aspects may be general to the organization and its function, others can be specific to a trial. It includes monitoring of process performance, implementation of any preventive or corrective action and change management. Performance indicators or metrics are measurable values of quality objectives and are an integral part of any quality system. As per regulations, upper management of an organization has the ultimate responsibility in the design, implementation and monitoring of a quality system.

Errors or deviations may potentially occur at any step of clinical trial operation, and these are called quality events. It may occur due to issues with the process, people, equipment, computerized system, or other reasons. The risk management strategy includes a system to document and investigate the quality events to establish the root causes and the contributory causes in a structured approach. Based on the investigations, corrections, corrective actions, and the preventive actions are taken. The criticality and impact of each quality event should be evaluated. As there can be many quality events occurring in an organization, it is triaged for necessary actions.

Root Cause Analysis (RCA) is necessary to determine the original or true cause of quality events. Corrections are immediate measures to secure a situation from the adverse impact of the quality events. Corrective actions are measures to prevent recurrence of such events, whereas preventive actions are measures to prevent potential quality events from occurring. Collectively, the acronym CAPA is used to describe the action plan in response to quality events. Every CAPA must be followed up for effectiveness over time by trend analysis.

As an example, the quality system in the context of informed consent form (ICF) development is described here. Typically, there are standard operating procedures (SOP) to develop an informed consent form as per the applicable guidance and regulation. The SOP identifies the roles and responsibilities of the persons involved. A checklist is used by another person to review the ICF for its conformity to good clinical practice (GCP) guideline as a quality control measure. A certain proportion of ICFs prepared by an organization can be randomly audited every year as a quality assurance procedure with a performance metric e.g. no ICF with deviation to GCP guidance.

A knowledge management system would ensure that the SOP and the checklist are updated as and when regulation or guideline changes. In case an audit or inspection finds an ICF to be incomplete despite the processes in place, it would be a quality event. In such a case, the quality risk management system would be utilized to investigate and recommend CAPAs. A performance metric can be devised to monitor that such deviation does not recur.

If this happens in the middle of a trial, the correction would be an immediate revision of the ICF and re- consent of the subjects. If it was found that the issues occurred due to the incomplete training of personnel, new training procedures may be devised to prevent recurrence of such ICF error as a corrective action. The preventive action may be to revisit the training procedure on other SOPs and implementation of a robust evaluation method for understanding following each training session.

Broadly, every organization involved in clinical trials such as the sponsor, clinical site, or clinical research organization (e.g. data management, statistics or monitoring) develops processes (SOPs, business guidance, and document templates) in accordance to regulations, guidance, standard scientific practice, and ethical principles with respect to their work. Each organization has a QA function to oversee development, review, and maintenance of processes and training of employees on that. Each individual is trained and is expected to follow the processes, protocol, or other trial documents for carrying out respective job on a day-to-day basis. Quality control measures are built around each major deliverable to ensure compliance to the respective processes or trial documents (e.g. protocol quality checklist, peer review of statistical analysis plan, or review of drug dispensing as per randomization list). Periodic audits are conducted by the QA function to ensure compliance with these processes and trial documents.

The processes and quality control methods are reviewed periodically to ensure alignment with applicable regulations. Sometimes, organizations appoint external agencies to audit internal processes for independent review (e.g. sponsor audit prior to regulatory submission of a dossier for product approval). In the addendum to ICH GCP guidance in 2016, a risk-based approach to quality management has been emphasized for implementation throughout all stages of a trial.

100. Standard operating procedure (SOP)

Standard operating procedure (SOP) is a written document outlining steps to perform a task or activity. The purpose of an SOP is to standardize a process, so that, the outcome is uniform and reproducible irrespective of the performer. In the context of clinical trials, SOPs are developed taking into consideration scientific principles, applicable regulations, ethical principles, and standard medical practice.

Many procedures in a clinical trial can be performed in several ways, and most of those might be acceptable as well; however, the outcome might not be consistent. For instance, blood pressure readings would be different depending on time, posture, place (arm or leg), the position of the manometer and reference point of the Korotkoff sound. Reproducible readings can only be obtained by following a process where these factors are uniform.

Each SOP typically has basic identification in the terms of the name of organization, number, the name of the procedure, personnel who have authored and approved its use, effective date, next date for revision, version control, changes to the previous version and reason for the change. In a complex environment, an SOP should identify the RACI matrix for the activity as far as possible.

RACI matrix:

- Responsible – The person who performs the activity
- Accountable – The person accountable to oversee the activity
- Consulted – The person who may be consulted in case of an exception
- Informed – The person who needs to be kept informed about the activity

Only important or key procedures should be governed by SOPs as too many SOPs may complicate routine function. It should be simple, flexible, feasible and in line with regulatory guidance as well as established scientific standards. There should be a reference to other related SOPs and forms that may be needed while performing an activity governed by an SOP. It is important to ensure that different SOPs are not in conflict with each other. Typically, there is a SOP to develop and maintain SOPs. In an organization involved in the clinical trial operation, there may be over a hundred SOPs, although not all may be relevant to each job function.

Regulatory authorities may review SOPs of an organization in the course of an inspection. Similarly, while outsourcing trial activities, sponsors would typically review SOPs of contract research organizations (CRO). Often, CROs are asked to follow sponsor's SOPs (e.g. trial monitoring or data management). In such cases, appropriate training needs to be provided to the identified personnel and documented before initiating any trial-related work.

During trial conduct, especially while a trial activity has been outsourced, there can be a conflict between the procedure in the protocol and the CRO SOP. Generally, the protocol supersedes the SOP and hence, the protocol should be followed. Sometimes, there could be conflicts between CRO and sponsor SOPs and it should be clarified.

Role-specific and activity-specific SOP training must be completed and documented before involvement in a trial. When sponsor's SOPs need to be followed, the staff at the CRO should be trained on those SOPs. Different modalities are available for SOP training and have been discussed separately.

SOP deviation may occur due to practical reasons, lack of awareness or inadequate training. It may be identified in routine monitoring, audits, or proactively by the study team. SOP deviations should be documented and the circumstance and its impact on the trial should be evaluated. Appropriate measures should be taken to prevent its recurrence. The quality assurance function plays a key role to formulate action plans to manage such issues.

SOPs are reviewed periodically to improve or change as per new regulation, scientific standard, practical consideration, or audit/inspection finding. If frequent SOP deviations are taking place for practical reasons, it should be reviewed from an operational perspective. Appropriate modifications may be considered and implemented within the acceptable scientific framework.

101. Training

Each clinical trial is different in terms of protocol and its implementation requirement. Variety of roles, responsibilities, and procedures come with each new clinical trial. Thus, personnel involved in trial conduct need to be trained appropriately to carry out their respective tasks effectively. The training may be on good clinical practice, standard operating procedures, software, devices, protocol, laboratory manual, or other topics as deemed relevant.

Training comprises of role and trial-specific training and is in addition to basic education or qualification. For instance, a registered pharmacist handles investigational product storage, dispensing, and subject randomization. An educational degree in pharmacy is the basic qualification. The pharmacist is further trained to work as a trial pharmacist. Additional study-specific training ensures that the pharmacist understands the requirements of a specific protocol. As per ICH GCP, each individual should be qualified by education, training, and experience to perform his or her respective task.

Organizations at all levels (e.g. sponsor, clinical site, and contract research organization) typically have a set of role-specific training modules related to their own business. These modules are on the general aspects of each roles; a person has to complete the specific module before taking up a particular role. If a person is responsible for multiple roles in a trial, there should be appropriate training for each of the role. In addition, each individual needs to be trained on the protocol and any other procedure specific to a particular trial.

Several methodologies are available for administering training such as instructor-led, self-reading or online. With advancement in information technology, most organizations are increasingly utilizing online digital platforms for role-specific training programmes with innovative audio and video content. Trial specific training could be administered in various ways depending on the specific need. For instance, protocol discussion could be in a face-to-face meeting, eCRF (case report form) training can be as an online training, while laboratory manual training can be as self-reading. It is a normal practice to assess understanding post training through some form of evaluation. At an organization level, there should be a mechanism of ongoing training to maximize effectiveness.

Training records are crucial documents in audits and inspections, and are often scrutinized. Role-specific and trial-specific training records can be maintained separately for convenience. While role-specific training records can be maintained in the personnel files of individual staff, trial-specific training records can be archived in the trial master file. With the increased use of digital platforms for training modules, the training completion can be automatically registered and a transcript can be retrieved from these portals as and when necessary.

102. Audit and inspection

Audit is defined in ICH GCP (good clinical practice) as 'a systematic and independent examination of trial related activities and documents to determine whether the evaluated trial related activities were conducted, and the data were recorded, analyzed and accurately reported according to the protocol, sponsor's standard operating procedures (SOPs), good clinical practice (GCP), and the applicable regulatory requirement(s).'

Inspection is defined in ICH GCP as 'the act by a regulatory authority(ies) of conducting an official review of documents, facilities, records, and any other resources that are deemed by the authority(ies) to be related to the clinical trial and that may be located at the site of the trial, at the sponsor's and/or CRO's (clinical research organization) facilities, or at other establishments deemed appropriate by the regulatory authority(ies).'

As evident in the definitions, the scope is quite wide in terms of activities and establishments that can come under the purview. Typically, an audit is conducted by the sponsor; additionally, sponsors or CROs may get their own work audited by an independent agency. For the sake of simplicity, this discussion is limited to audit or inspection of a clinical site.

Audit and inspection are integral components of the clinical trial process, and are not exceptional events. It can happen at any time before, during, or after the trial. The reasons are broadly either routine or for-cause. A sponsor may routinely audit certain trials (randomly selected or crucial trials) as a quality assurance measure. Audits planned in reaction to suspected irregularities are called 'for-cause' audits. Inspections may have similar reasons.

Health authorities may routinely inspect a certain proportion of trials as a policy. For-cause inspection may be initiated for important trials related to a product approval or in response to suspected irregularities, (e.g. notification from sponsor about misconduct, an investigator conducting too many trials, there is suspicious data or inconsistencies). Trials for regulatory submission are more likely to be inspected than others since marketing authorization depend on it. These studies are also frequently audited by the sponsors by own quality assurance department or independent agencies to ensure appropriate study conduct and to prepare the sites for possible inspection.

While both audit and monitoring are conducted by the sponsor, there are differences between these two activities. Monitor is part of the trial team, and proactively partners with the site in trial conduct. Monitoring takes place while the study is ongoing, therefore, errors can be identified and rectified in a timely manner. The monitor has a responsibility to work with the site to ensure trial conduct as per expectations. In contrast, an audit is a retrospective verification of compliance, and the auditors are independent of the trial team. Auditors have no such responsibility or mandate to work with the trial team for compliance. Little can be done to the trial conduct when findings are identified in the audit process late in the trial conduct or after completion.

An audit assists the sponsor to independently evaluate the trial, and take preventive or corrective measures if necessary; auditors have no authority to take any legal action but to only report to the sponsor or any other party who instituted the audit (e.g. CRO) about the findings. On the other hand, inspections are conducted by empowered authorities, and they have powers to take legal actions in case of deviations.

The basic process of audit and inspection is similar. Typically, a schedule is informed in advance; however, inspections may occur without prior notice depending on the situation. It begins with an introductory meeting followed by review of trial conduct, which comprises of facility tour, a review of documents as well as an interview of the staff and investigator. This is followed by a closing meeting. The duration may range from one day to several days depending on the scope.

In the introductory meeting, the auditors/inspectors outline the purpose and scope of the audit/inspection. The clinical site may brief about the organization, facility, organogram and the personnel who would assist in the process. In the closing meeting, the findings are discussed; it is also an opportunity to clarify any point, which has been misunderstood.

The objective of any audit or inspection is to verify compliance with standard processes and identify irregularities. Auditors and inspectors generally try to reconstruct the sequence of events in the study conduct. Review of records, interview with staff and facility visit are the usual methods. Site staff may be asked to demonstrate certain procedures. Inspectors may carry back documents, IP (investigational product) samples, or devices for further investigation; however, this would not be the case in an audit. Here are the typical trial activities that frequently come under scrutiny.

- Trial timelines and sequence of events
- Ethics committee (EC) approval of protocols, amendments and informed consent forms (ICF); EC notifications and communications

- Delegation of activities, supervision by investigator, training and qualification of staff, training by sponsor and process to ensure adequate training
- Method of recruitment, informed consent process, and enrolment
- Method of entry criteria verification and assessment of safety/efficacy endpoints
- Adverse event identification, documentation, and reporting
- IP shipment, storage, disposition, retrieval or destruction
- Monitoring process
- Trial data collection, documentation, reporting and archival
- Compliance with protocol and SOPs
- Financial interests of investigator and site staff
- Adequacy of facility and resource for trial conduct
- Investigator file, protocol, organogram, SOPs, CV of personnel, training records, and quality manual

The site should identify a lead, preferably from quality assurance function to coordinate between the auditors/inspectors and the internal stakeholders. In the event of an inspection, the clinical site should also notify the sponsor. There could be legal considerations while complying with requests from inspectors as per regulations. Clarity on those aspects from company's legal counsel is helpful. Following are a few points on the general approach to face audit/inspection.

- Clinical sites should have an SOP to handle audit/inspection
- Internal or independent audit may be conducted periodically to familiarize with the process
- Clinical trial documents should be regularly updated as a policy
- Once the audit/inspection is scheduled, the scope and timeframe should be clarified with the sponsor or the authorities
- Responsibilities of individual staff should be identified and discussed
- Site staff should review the protocol and their individual responsibilities in the particular trial

- Prior to the scheduled day, preparedness should be reviewed by the lead in the form of a mock run
- In the introductory meeting, the plan of audit/inspection should be clarified including personnel to be interviewed and documents to be reviewed
- Auditors and inspectors should be accompanied at all times and should not be left alone except upon their request
- Staff should be specific and to the point to requests/questions. The focus should be on the current audit/inspection. Unsolicited questions, responses, or descriptions should be avoided.
- All requested documents should be readily made available. If copies of documents are requested, it should be provided marking as 'copy' and documented.
- Staff should be confident, polite, and cooperative. Any identified true deficiency should be readily acknowledged without arguments
- Closing meeting is crucial to clarify any misunderstanding of issues

In due course, the inspection report is communicated to the investigator or sponsor. The format and process may vary depending on the health authority. For instance, US FDA provides an initial classification of the inspection based on the observations noted during the inspection as NAI (no action indicated i.e. no findings), VAI (voluntary action indicated i.e. informational) or OAI (official action indicated i.e. warning). Generally, the investigator/sponsor would have an opportunity to respond with clarification or planned and implemented action. This process can continue until resolution of the issues, legal action, or further inspection. Inspection finding of high public interest may be posted in public domain as per country regulation.

The implications of inspection finding could be warning to take corrective measures or legal actions including criminal proceedings in extreme cases. The investigator could be disqualified to carry out any future trial; the sponsor might have implications in terms of delay in approval or rejection of the marketing application.

In case of an audit, the report is submitted to the sponsor, who in turn discusses the findings with the investigator. The sponsor may also work with the site to devise an action plan. The agreed measures to be taken as well as those already implemented should be documented. In extreme cases, the site may be terminated. As indicated earlier, auditors per se have no authority and any such action has to be taken by the sponsor.

Here are the commonly observed findings in audits/inspections:

- Protocol deviations
- Noncompliance with adverse event reporting
- Failure to report concomitant therapy
- Inadequate and inaccurate records
- Issues with EC procedures, approvals, and communications
- Issues with the informed consent documents or process
- Issues with IP accountability

The response plan to audit or inspection findings are described in the form of CAPA (Corrective Actions and Preventive Actions) i.e. a systematic approach that includes actions needed to correct (correction), avoid re-occurrence (corrective action), and eliminate the cause of potential quality issues (preventive action). Corrections or remedial measures are taken as one-time fixes for immediate solutions.

For instance, if protocol deviations have occurred in a trial due to errors in a site SOP, a memo identifying the error in the SOP with an instruction to follow a correct procedure would be the correction. An amendment to the SOP would be a corrective action and be developing a robust review process to prevent such errors in SOPs would be a preventive action.

The audit/inspection readiness is a concept of managing audits and inspections in the regulated environment of clinical research. It is a holistic approach comprising of awareness and trial conduct in compliance to applicable regulations, preparation for audit/inspection, handling questions during audit/inspection as well as taking appropriate actions based on the findings.

103. Misconduct or fraud in clinical trial

Clinical trials must be conducted as per the protocol, good clinical practice (GCP), standard operating procedures, applicable regulations, and ethical principles. Crucial decisions are taken on safety/efficacy of investigational products based on clinical trial data. Stakeholders may violate these basic principles for vested interests leading to trial misconduct. Instances of misconduct have been reported in the literature and are not uncommon, and it can have serious implications on the trial validity.

Clinical research misconduct is defined by US FDA as falsification of data in proposing, processing, designing, performing, recording, supervising, reviewing, analyzing, collecting clinical research, or reporting clinical research results, outcomes and endpoints. Although exact figure on fraud or misconduct is difficult to ascertain, it may not be so unusual to discover a trial affected by some form of fraud or misconduct in a person's career.

US FDA uses the terminology 'fraud' and 'misconduct' interchangeably. It can be an act of 'omission' i.e. consciously not revealing all data or an act of 'commission' i.e. consciously altering or fabricating data. Fraud does not include honest error or honest difference in opinion. Deliberate or repeated noncompliance with the protocol and GCP is considered fraud. Generally, data falsification is taken more seriously and has severe implications.

Here are few examples of misconduct observed by health authorities (HA):

Clinical Investigators

- Mismatch of time suggesting fraud
- Failure to maintain adequate and accurate case histories
- Falsification of laboratory reports
- Failure to adequately supervise the trial

Sponsors/contract research organizations

- Inadequate documentation of study personnel selection
- Inadequate monitoring of the trial
- Improper investigator selection

Ethics committees (EC)

- Inadequate or improper review of the research proposal
- Failure to ensure a reasonably informed consent form

All parties involved in clinical research can potentially get involved in misconduct or fraud. Several factors such as financial gains, desire to progress in career, overwork, conflicts of interest, reputational gain and achievement with less effort are typical motivations for fraudulent activities. A general level of awareness, vigilance, and systematic approach is required at all level to sense and prevent trial misconduct. Notably, clinical sites are often implicated in trial misconduct.

The field monitor is at the forefront when it comes to the detection of fraud at clinical sites. With access to all documents at the clinical site and periodic face-to-face interaction with site personnel during onsite visits, the monitor can sense any fraudulent behavior at the site. A careful review of source data provides an opportunity to verify data integrity. Cross verification of data from different sources (appointment diaries, logbook, lab report, clinic notes, etc) to reconstruct the sequence of events could be a powerful method to detect fraud.

Monitors may be alerted in situations with alteration in source data, missing subject identifiers in laboratory reports, too perfect subject diary entry, similarity in the handwriting of different subjects, too perfect drug accountability, non-availability of trial documentation in time for monitoring, frequent postponement of monitoring visits, absence of trial staff during visits, and low incidence of screen failure or adverse event. The monitors should be given free hand to investigate and report any misconduct to the sponsor. There are instances of clinical site staff turning whistleblowers and reporting issues to authorities.

Misconduct could be identified by careful review of trial data, and it has become easier due to electronic format of reporting as well as access to analytics tools. Data review may indicate unusual trends at a particular site. Protocol non-compliance can be reflected in the laboratory evaluation of biomarkers. Digit preferences may be evident when data has been manipulated or created.

Considering the wide scope of misconduct, the difficulty to detect when done in a subtle way, and the serious consequences, everyone involved in trials has a responsibility to prevent it. Good documentation practice, systematically planned verification, appropriate training, quality control measures, zero tolerance policy, whistle-blower protection, a clear policy to handle such situations, and promotion of model ethical behavior are certain ways to discourage such activities. Once there is suspicion of possible fraudulent activity, an investigation must be initiated. After a preliminary review, a for-cause audit may be initiated.

Organizations should have SOPs to manage such situations; staff should be trained on the overall approach and their individual roles. The scope includes initial action upon suspicion, escalation and communication procedure, confidentiality, investigation requirement, evidence preservation, reporting responsibility (e.g. to management, regulatory authorities, ethics committee) and whistleblower protection. Sponsors are expected to report promptly any such suspicion involving trial data to the HAs and ECs as required per local regulations.

In a situation of trial misconduct at a clinical site, the action plan would largely depend on the nature of the misconduct and its potential impact. It might be possible to salvage the situation through training as well as creating awareness among the investigator and site staff about the implications. Monitoring efforts may be intensified for close supervision. Any identified misconduct must be documented, and quality assurance department should be consulted while dealing with such a situation. Deliberate non-compliance in spite of repeated training and awareness efforts should be documented before declaring it as misconduct.

Termination of the site could be considered for situations, which cannot be salvaged or are of serious in nature. EC/HA should be notified as per local regulations. Participating subjects may be transferred to nearby trial sites if possible; else, subjects could be withdrawn from the trial as per the protocol and managed with standard of care in the locality. Handling the data from such a site (i.e. suspected of trial misconduct) is usually questionable. The choices are either analysis after exclusion of the suspicious data or presentation of the data with a sensitivity analysis (including and excluding the suspicious data).

Trial misconduct at any level potentially affects data integrity and raises several questions on the trial validity as well as individuals and organizations involved in the trial. The reputation of organizations built over years may be tarnished due to vested interests of few individuals. Misconduct may never be eliminated; however, the scale of it can be significantly minimized by a systematic proactive approach. Each individual at every level of trial conduct has a responsibility to prevent it.

104. Trial risk mitigation plan

The clinical phase of drug development is a complex interdependent activity, and timely completion of clinical trials is critical for swift decision-making or timely market access. The trial operation, similar to any other large project with considerable dependencies, could be derailed to deliver quality results or meet timelines with considerable impact on downstream planning. A risk mitigation plan (RMP) essentially identifies risk factors and lines up strategies to handle adverse situations.

'Risk' is a commonly used term in clinical trials in the context of the safety of subjects and quality of trial conduct. Risk-benefit assessment is the fundamental consideration before allowing any clinical trial for a society. A risk-based approach to quality management at all stages of trial conduct has been advised in the ICH-GCP guidance. The objective of the present topic is a bit different in a sense that it is focussed on the big picture of deliverables from a trial. One of the basic expectations of various stakeholders from a clinical trial project manager is continuous assessment of risk factors and proactive planning to manage that.

Both internal and external factors can be risks to trial conduct. Examples of internal factors are lack of budget commitment, non-availability of trial drugs or delay in protocol development. Examples of external factors can be regulatory hurdles, recruitment issues, difficulty in protocol implementation, vendor-related issues or competing trials.

RMP should be developed carefully taking into consideration these factors, its implications, potential ways to mitigate it or contingency plan if a risk materializes. Often, RMP is a living and informal document and is updated periodically (e.g. every month and prior to important milestones such as trial initiation). Individual functions identify the risks, likely impact, mitigation plan, contingency plan, and the stakeholders responsible to monitor and take necessary action. A scoring methodology could be used to quantify the risk in terms of probability of occurrence and its likely impact although it could be very subjective.

The complexity of RMP depends on the magnitude and complexity of the trials. The risks identified should be practical and based on real-life experiences or reasonable possibilities rather than entirely hypothetical situations. The RMP helps to create best and worst-case scenarios for the stakeholders. It creates awareness of the practical realities and prepares the team to anticipate and cope with situations. The RMP should be discussed with the relevant stakeholders to evaluate preparedness as well as to sensitize the possibilities and backup strategies. There should be a mechanism to feed into the risks at the program level from individual studies.

105. Ethical and legal aspects in clinical trial

Clinical trials present a complex problem to the human society. While it is unequivocal that these are necessary, the best way to run this in the most acceptable way is still debated. Ethics is a set of moral principles to guide and determine what is right or wrong, whereas law is the system of rules to enforce the right behavior. A detailed discussion on this topic is beyond the scope of this discussion. However, the topic is briefly introduced in the context of trial operations.

Ethical aspects:

The broader ethical principles, which govern human experimentation, are respect for fellow humans, beneficence, and justice. Many of the ethical rules originate from these basic principles. Here are some of those relevant ethical rules.

- Scientific validity and social value: Any potential human experimentation must have scientific validity with a clear objective, an answerable question, and robust methodology. The answer to the research question should add value to further health so that it justifies exposing subjects to the risk.

- Respect for subjects: It guides the treatment of subjects without prejudice at all times irrespective of their decision. Essential elements are a provision of adequate information, autonomy, privacy, confidentiality, due care, and safety measures.

- Risk-benefit paradigm: The risk to subjects should be minimized. Risks can be physical, mental, social, or financial. When the anticipated risk exceeds the anticipated benefit, the experiment must stop. Trials in healthy subjects pose a challenge as no benefit is anticipated and hence, there has to be low tolerance to any anticipated risk.

- Informed consent: The subjects must be free to exercise autonomy in participation as well as a continuation of participation without prejudice. There are two components to it. The subjects should get all relevant information about risk, benefit, methodology, options, any new information, and then take decisions voluntarily without any influence. In situations, when a subject may not be in a position to make a decision, a proxy may be empowered for decision making consistent with the subject's values and interests.

- Fair selection: The approach to enrol subjects should be based only on scientific objective and not on vulnerability, privilege or any other reason. Every eligible subject should get an opportunity to make an informed choice. Those who make this choice should get the benefit and share any burden or risk associated with the experiment.

- Indemnification for injury: The subjects participating in trials should be taken care of and compensated for any injury due to the experimentation.

- Conflicts of interest: Any human experimentation proposal should be reviewed independently without bias for the ethical aspects before and during the conduct. This is typically done by health authorities, ethics committees, and in some cases to some extent by data safety monitoring boards.

Legal aspects:

Specific rules and regulations govern clinical trial conduct in each country e.g. schedule Y of drugs and cosmetic act and rules in India. There is a clear legal obligation for compliance with such regulations. Additionally, several national and international guidelines (e.g. ICH-GCP) need be complied with for trial conduct. Many other regulations have indirect implications for clinical trials. Here are some examples:

- Confidentiality and privacy rules (e.g. HIPAA in the US)
- Regulations for practice of medicine
- Regulations for medical negligence
- Compensation for injury
- Regulations for indemnities
- Regulations on human rights
- Fraud or professional misconduct
- Regulations for biological sample management
- Regulations for handling drugs in the country
- Intellectual property rules
- Publication rights

There are reports of litigations in the context of clinical trials involving allegations such as inadequate information about risks, improper informed consent, research misconduct, conflicts of interest, and violations of basic ethical principles. Any of the involved parties i.e. investigator, institution, ethics committee, and sponsor can be implicated in such litigations.

One a day today basis many situations warrant legal consultations e.g. compensation to investigators or subjects, purchase of equipment for sites, consent form text, protocol provisions, advertisement texts, clinical trial disclosures, trial insurance, indemnity provisions, contracts, etc. Legal compliance is a standard component of review for many trial documents.

106. Information technology systems in clinical trial

Widespread use of computers and IT systems has led to a transformation in the way organizations operate. This is also true for clinical research industry with the availability of new platform technologies. Rules, regulations, and guidance are under continuous revision to accommodate such changes. Processes related to trial planning, operation, project management, communication, document management and data handling have undergone significant transformation.

Penetration of IT system use varies among organizations, and from one activity to another in the same organization. IT systems have enabled more flexibility, automation, remote work environment while reducing paperwork and accelerating processes. Mobile and cloud-based platforms are further transforming the IT-enabled environment.

Various IT-enabled tools are now commonly in use for trial planning and project management. Web-based platforms are available for site identification, budget estimation, timelines planning and risk identification. Integration of data from various IT systems such as Clinical Trial Management System (CTMS), Interactive Response Technologies (IRT), Trial Supply Chain

Management (SCM) System, Electronic Data Capture (EDC) is a powerful approach that provides ready access to trial related information on a real-time basis and in intuitive dashboards. Built-in programs in databases are increasingly in use for event-triggered notifications.

Electronic document management system is now common for trial-related document management. Document creation, edition, version control, publication, and archival are routinely managed in electronic formats. It supports features such as remote access, controlled access, audit trail, version control, recovery in case of accidental modification or deletion. Documents can be approved and signed off electronically in such systems and it reduces the need for paper copies and physical movements. Health authorities and ethics committees increasingly require dossiers in electronic formats to reduce the paper load. Routine interaction with authorities such as trial applications and approvals are taking place online. A gradual shift is taking place to archive trial documents in an electronic trial master file.

Emails and instant messaging are the most common mode of communication due to the inherent advantages. Customized communication platforms are now available for responding to site questions. Automated communication systems are increasingly used to send event notifications, milestone updates, and reminders. SharePoint is in use as interfaces for information and document sharing. Internet-based web meetings with capabilities for audio, video and document sharing are fast replacing in person or telephonic meetings.

Most organizations currently administer training through interactive web-based platforms. Features such as individualized assignment, remote access, and audio/video content are common along with several other customizable features. Understanding of training can be simultaneously evaluated with innovative methods that document training completion automatically. Such platforms allow on-demand access to training as well as remote monitoring of training completion.

The subject recruitment process is changing with the advent of social media. Advertisement of clinical trials over social media is allowed in certain countries. It is typically easy to find the target audience and advocacy groups in such online forums, especially for rare diseases. Biometric systems are in use in some places to prevent cross participation in clinical trials. Web-based IRT systems are the preferred modality for randomization and treatment allocation. Investigators' portals are in use to communicate with multiple investigators, share documents, and update trial progress.

Subject data can be directly captured in electronic source documents at the clinical sites. Mobile applications are available to directly collect patient-reported outcome data, set up reminders for subjects or as communication tools. Wearable devices that can measure and transmit body parameters online on a real-time basis are increasing under evaluation. Remote tracking of sample movement, remote access of laboratory data (such as hematology, biochemistry, ECG, imaging, pulmonary function) and swift transfer of such data to trial databases are the new norm.

Remote and electronic web-based systems are the preferred mode in data management. Software use is the norm in the next steps of data analysis and reporting. Newer techniques of remote monitoring and data analytics have enabled a targeted and risk-based approach to monitoring. Specialized software programs are in use for safety data management and reporting to authorities.

Security of the IT systems is a major concern. The security measures include both physical and logical measures such as controlled access, passwords, secured networks, anti-virus programs, proper locking of the computer systems and so on. Processes are built to allow use by authorized personnel for the designated purpose only. The possibility of data loss and breach of privacy regulations are other sensitive topics in the IT-enabled milieu.

System dependability must be verifiable through validation, and documented. The software and other computer systems must be validated, and any change implementation should be controlled and documented. While developing new programs, testing is a key component, which must be undertaken by the developer, quality control personnel, and the end user. User acceptance testing is a step in which the end users have an opportunity to evaluate the system before the program goes into production.

There should be written standard operating procedures to handle contingencies. Proper methods must be available for data backup, recovery, and alternate means in case of system failure. Data loss in case of natural calamities is a huge threat. Integrity and preparedness must be evaluated through audit and stress testing. Many of these systems and applications also depend on the high-speed internet to access database servers and it must be ensured.

Currently, IT platforms are in use in every step of clinical research, and the use is rapidly increasing due to the convenience it offers. Familiarity with computer and IT systems is now essential for any job function in this field. Processes and practices to ensure proper and safe use of IT systems are critical.

107. Interactive voice, web or mobile response technology (IRT)

IRT is a technology solution used in several industries for managing automated interactions that involve simple input and output of data. The clinical trial industry has adopted it to support some of the processes related to enrolment, randomization, investigational product (IP) dispensing, inventory management of trial supply, and subject visit tracking. Integration of IRT to other technology tools and data capture systems works as a force multiplier in trial information management.

In the voice format, a person dials a telephone number and inputs data using telephone keypad in response to pre-recorded voice prompts. The required output information is provided through fax or email to pre-identified authorized personnel. In the web or mobile format, such information transaction takes place in the web or mobile interface.

Typical input info is country, site number, subject identifiers (e.g. date of birth, gender, initial), visit name, visit date, subject status (e.g. visit completed, screened failed, early terminated, a study completed), or medication number (e.g. received shipment number, quarantined medication number). Typical output info is subject number, confirmation of subject status, successful recording of trial data, medication number assigned, or treatment group allocation. Programming of databases enables transaction of such information and it can be customized to the need.

The need for an IRT is considered on a case-by-case basis for individual trials. While it is indispensable in a multicounty multicentre randomized blinded trial, it is not essential in an open level trial with a few sites. Here are some of the common uses of IRT:

Enrolment and randomization:

- Randomization to different study arms
- Complex stratified randomizations to ensure random equal allocation of subjects to different sub-groups in the study between different treatment groups e.g. age-groups, region, disease severity or gender
- Manage enrolment distribution by limiting enrolment of subjects with specific characteristics e.g. disease severity, country, and age-group

Real-time subject status summary:

- Screened, screen failure, reason for screen failure, randomized, visit completion, trial completion, withdrawal

- Study, country, and site level summary of subject status

IP dispensing and inventory management:

- Dispensing uniquely numbered IP packs (specific to randomized treatment group allocation or other predefined characteristics)
- Dispensing in the order of expiry date
- Manual or automated resupply requests to IP distribution depot once site inventory is below certain threshold
- Efficient management of inventory as well as future prediction of medication usage involving complex situations such as IP with short shelf life, temperature excursions making IP unusable, rapidly changing recruitment or subject withdrawal
- IP Inventory management and paperless accountability documentation through electronic tracking of each pack from packaging through central depot, local depot, study site until use, destruction, or retrieval

Blinding and emergency code breaks:

- Maintain blinding in blinded trials
- Allow unblinding by authorized personnel in emergency situations

Patient Reported Outcome (PRO) data collection, reminders, and notifications:

- Collection of outcome measures directly from trial subjects
- Remind subjects and site staff about upcoming visits
- Event triggered notifications to study personnel e.g. unblinding, termination

Recruitment management:

- Administration of pre-screening questionnaires to potential subjects approaching through toll-free numbers or trial web portals in response to advertisements

- Management of screening appointments at the nearest study site
- Assess effectiveness of advertisement campaigns

IRT portals are programmed to generate customized reports tailored to users. Blinded and unblinded users at both sponsor and site level can obtain a summary or detailed reports with information about the sites, subject visits, IP inventory, IP distribution status, etc. Access to the different reports is configured at the time of IRT setup. It is customized to the user profile and can be changed as needed.

Several IT applications are in use for efficient management of clinical trials. It is recognized that the true potential of these applications can be realized by integration of all the applications such as IRT, Clinical Trial Management System (CTMS), Drug Supply Management System (DSMS) and Electronic Data Capture (EDC) system.

Most of these systems are data hungry, and certain systems have more real-time data than others (e.g. IRT vs. EDC) do. Each system can feed data to other systems to minimize manual efforts in data entry while improving accuracy and bringing automation. For example, when a site is created within CTMS, it can create a new site in IRT, which in turn can feed subject data to EDC once a new subject is enrolled.

108. Clinical trial management system (CTMS)

Project managers need a considerable amount of information about the clinical sites, vendors, trial documents, site activation, recruitment, invoice payment, IP supply, site monitoring, etc. for efficient management of trials and review of its progress. The stakeholders involved in trial conduct need such information for planning their work. Conventionally, project managers manually collect and track such information using spreadsheets, paper logs and so on. However, such manual approach is highly inefficient, time-consuming and unfriendly with the propensity for errors or duplication of efforts.

Clinical Trial Management System (CTMS) is a customizable technology solution to manage incredible amount operational information from various sources to help in planning and managing clinical trials. Several such commercial applications are available, and many sponsors or CROs have developed such applications for in-house use. While requirements are broadly similar, there could be subtle differences that need customization. All trial-related information relevant for assessing trial process and efficient oversight of site activities, budget and compliance are the requirements.

CTMS depends on the prompt availability of data, which is either reported by field monitors, site personnel, vendors, project managers or populated from other trial databases such as IRT, EDC, eTMF, and invoice management systems. Integration of the different databases is necessary for the seamless flow of information. Reports on high-level metrics can be visualized in interactive dashboards as graphs or tables with a capability to drill down to desired levels (e.g. trial, country, site, or individual subject). Typically, such applications are supported by analytics algorithms to generate the desired metrics.

Typical reports of interest are about EC or HA submission activities, approvals, start-up activities, contracts, site activation, subject visits, monitoring visits, monitoring findings, protocol deviations, recruitment progress, quality metrics, invoice payments, site closeout activities, trial milestones, etc. Under each category, various predefined metrics can be estimated e.g. summary of regulatory approvals, import/export licenses obtained, source data verification completed, pending invoices, sites with slow recruitment, data management queries, etc. Such information is periodically necessary and is difficult to compile manually in larger trials.

CTMS configuration is needed at the beginning of a trial for unique requirements. It is primarily driven by the desirability of the reports, metrics and the information feeding mechanisms. For instance, granular information about enrolment, subject status or data management in the trial can be obtained by integrating to IRT or EDC databases. Integration of trial supply management systems, eTMF, payment systems, and safety reporting systems can provide additional data to the system. Certain information may still need to be manually entered if it cannot be fetched from other systems (e.g. site contact details, EC submission status, approval availability, contract execution, site activation, monitoring visits).

CTMS can complement site monitoring activities. Updates for monitoring visit preparation and visit report generation can be obtained from CTMS while key updates from the visit reports can feed data to CTMS. Gradually, electronic monitoring visit reports integrated to CTMS are becoming the norm.

Summaries of subject status, protocol deviation (PD), source data verification, or list of subjects monitored (based on subject visits completed until a particular visit) can be auto-populated to the visit report from CTMS, while updates about any significant findings, issues that are open or closed in the visit, submission of documents to EC (e.g. PD list, SUSARs), site payment status, changes to site staff, etc. can be automatically extracted to CTMS from the visit reports. The open items in a monitoring visit can be auto-populated in the next visit report for follow up.

CTMS is indispensable to project managers for managing large multicounty and multicentre trials. Operational information can be retrieved instantly to update stakeholders or review of trial progress. Key issues and roadblocks can be identified and tracked efficiently for resolution without the need for manual tracking. At an organization level, CTMS can provide an overview of all ongoing clinical trials. It can also serve as an effective interface for sponsors to oversee outsourced trials.

109. Electronic document management system

Enormous numbers of documents are generated and need to be archived to support audit trail of trial activities. In a large phase 3 trial, tens of thousands of documents could be generated. With an increase in the number of trials, globalization of both the trials and teams managing it, and the need to archive documents for a long duration, there is a natural trend to move to a paperless environment. As such, the transition to a paperless environment has taken place across organizations directly or indirectly involved in clinical trials. Regulatory acceptance of electronic documents and widespread use of computer systems and web applications have helped this change.

Documents could be in various forms and generated in different circumstances by parties directly or indirectly involved in the trial. The protocol, investigator's brochure, and ICF are used by the trial team and clinical sites to conduct the trial, obtain subject consent or review of the trial proposal by authorities. Subject medical records such as the patient file, lab reports, ECG strips or imaging films are generated part of medical care but also serve as source documents. Manuals on pharmacy, laboratory, or IRT are typically prepared to guide sites about study procedures. Audio/video materials are used for advertisement or site training. Airway bills, temperature logs, and invoices are generated during trial material supply to trial sites. Approvals and permissions are obtained from authorities to allow trial conduct or trial supply.

Electronic document management systems address some of the common expectations such as collaborative authoring, content management, ownership, accountability, audit trail, legibility, remote access, controlled access, security, encryption, and compliance to privacy or confidentiality regulations, archival in a specific structure, ability to search documents and system backup. It can be configured to manage specific requirement of each type of document.

Certain documents (e.g. study report) need an environment for authoring, review, approval by a team and publishing, while others (e.g. regulatory approval) are externally final documents, and only need to be uploaded to the system for archival. Dossiers for authorities need complex publishing step involving elaborate electronic index and link creation for the necessary set of documents. Quality control steps are incorporated into the individual document lifecycle as necessary.

Some organizations have developed own systems while others use licensed systems from service providers. Familiarity with navigation and folder structure within such systems requires both training and experience. Electronic systems have been developed primarily targeting two locations where trial documents are primarily created or archived i.e. sponsor's Trial Master File (TMF) and Investigator's TMF (or Investigator's File). Many other associated functions of the sponsor (e.g. clinical development, discovery, CMC and regulatory) are also involved in document management, and the system usually supports various documents managed by all stakeholders of the sponsor with an overarching structure. This is particularly important for the regulatory function that communicates with authorities or makes dossier submission. Such systems also help to keep a track of all external submissions.

Currently, guidance from major regulatory authorities is available on expected standards of electronic TMF (eTMF) to promote a paperless direction. However, full clarity on the acceptability of a fully paperless system is lacking and is a potential residual risk. Issues about scanning standards and its QC process, compatibility issues of storage media after a long time with the then current systems, and storage media lifespan are some of the key concerns. Many organizations have adopted a dual strategy to either keep documents in both formats or minimize paper formats to the extent possible.

The newer approach to eTMF envisages having an integrated system where all stakeholders such as a sponsor, CRO, and clinical sites can create, manage, and share documents in a controlled environment. It would obviate the need for manual sharing of documents while enabling quicker access to current versions and improving compliance. Standardized document naming convention and folder structure would allow oversight of completeness though visualization of metrics in a dashboard. The system could flag noncompliance and remind stakeholders of necessary action.

110. Trial supply chain management system

Clinical trial supplies to the clinical sites include investigational medicinal products, laboratory kits, devices or equipment, ancillary supplies, and documents. Clinical sites usually send clinical samples, digital media, images, and documents (e.g. patient files for adjudication committee) to central/regional facilities for further processing, analysis, or storage. Unused supplies not meant for local disposition are retrieved from the clinical sites.

Electronic systems are often used for managing such supplies especially in large global multicounty trials. Different supplies may be managed separately by functions or vendors and may have its own specific requirements e.g. logistic of IP supply could be quite different from a lab supply. Specific requirements are well known, and it is considered in trial planning. Following are some of the common expectations in terms of capabilities of electronic systems supporting trial supplies:

- Country regulations: Import and export licenses are typically required at country or state entry or exit points. The regulations vary from country to country and may change over time. A quickly accessible central repository of such information is helpful for supply chain experts.

- Integration to other tools: Clinical trial management system (CTMS), interactive response technology (IRT) and electronic data capture (EDC) are an integral part of trial operations. Once integrated, such tools can seamlessly share relevant information for best function (e.g. country and site list, project milestones, number of subjects for each site, upcoming visit for individual subjects, etc).

- Forecasting and overage estimation: The system could auto calculate and forecast requirements taking into consideration enrolment projection and overages based on inbuilt logics and inputs from other tools. This could be further auto adjusted as the trial progresses.

- Packaging and labelling considerations: There is specific packaging and labelling requirements for individual countries, and the system should be able to auto suggest the needs. For example, packaging standards could vary depending on geographic location and season.

- Storage and distribution network mapping: Trial supplies are stored at central and local depots to help quicker delivery to trial sites. Many organizations have regional hubs or country depots as intermediaries besides central hubs.

- Clinical site storage capacity: Sites may be conducting many clinical trials with different sponsors besides their own research. Availability of environment and access controlled space is a key factor often overlooked and may be limited for individual trials. For example, storage area in nitrogen tank for laboratory samples or 2-8 0C refrigerators for IP may be limited.

- Request and supply delivery process: It could be automated or managed manually in the electronic system. Typically, processes exist for initial supply (triggered by site activation), re-supply request, cancellation of supply request, supply receipt confirmation as well as notification of any damaged or quarantined supply, etc. It is important to understand how these requests are linked to downstream activities of the shipper (e.g. lead-time for delivery, picking up a supply, intermediate storage, customs clearance, transport, etc).

- Inventory visibility: Electronic systems integrated with other clinical trial tools such as IRT, CTMS, and EDC help in assessing inventory of supplies to and from the sites at various locations including the clinical sites. This insight is necessary to trigger resupply or minimize wastage.

- Shipment frequency determination: Multitude of factors such as storage capacity, feasibility, cost, and other specific requirements determine shipment frequency. For instance, biological samples may have to be shipped weekly due to storage capacity limitation at the site, stability considerations or capacity issues at the analytical laboratories. The frequency of drug supplies may be decided by storage capacity, the pace of enrolment and shelf life.

- Unusable trial supply management: Visibility of unusable supplies in the inventory is necessary for accountability and for the ability to quarantine, destroy or retrieve from the clinical sites. Clear processes must be built in to alert such instances and trigger next processes.

- Tracking, reconciliation, and accountability: Ability to locate not only shipments but also each individual unit (e.g. laboratory kit, laboratory sample or IP kit) is necessary. It is often necessary to fast-track a sample analysis or exclude a certain IP kit from dispensing. Accountability of IP, trial supplies and reconciliation of samples received at central labs are standard requirements. Logics could be built in to enable smooth transportation, tracking, and reconciliation. Barcodes or microchips simplify tracking and electronic reconciliation procedures.

- Supply risk identification: Ability to maintain optimum inventory at the sites must be ensured through timely supply, waste minimization and risk flagging of supply run outs.

- Reports: Generation of summary and detailed reports at various levels such as trial, region, country, and site for status metrics are necessary to understand the status.

111. Clinical trials and media

Clinical trials may draw the attention of traditional and social media in a positive or negative way. There is a considerable suspicion of clinical trials due to historical anecdotes of unethical practices. As such, considerable prejudice is not unusual about drug trials and pharmaceutical companies conducting such trial for product development. Media stories and social media talking points may whip up public sentiments that may disrupt trial operations. While positive reports of the contribution of clinical trials to healthcare may not be uncommon, the theme could often be of exploitation.

Adverse events, compensation in clinical trials, consent process, the inclusion of vulnerable subjects (e.g. children), trial outcomes, for-cause inspection by authorities, or trial misconduct are the typical topics that draw media attention. As such, there could be rumors that become media stories and further complicate the situation due to a spread of misinformation. Fundamentally, it could vitiate the trust between investigators and trial subjects. New subjects may hesitate to enrol while already enrolled subjects may be disturbed to continue participation. It could evoke considerable attention from authorities trying to manage the situation. Besides, investigators and subjects, other stakeholders such as CRO partners may be affected.

While any trial could be the point of discussion, certain trials are more likely to draw such attention. A vulnerable population, delicate risk-benefit profile, and scale of trial are the usual considerations. Proactive planning is helpful to prevent chaos during trial conduct. External agencies may be hired to support media management.

A media management plan could be developed to identify roles and responsibilities. The media management plan includes training of stakeholders, preparing reactive statements, monitoring of media including social media, assessing any situations, which may become media stories, responding to media questions and developing strategies to reassure stakeholders.

Any person at the sponsor or partner organization and a clinical site may be contacted by journalists. There should be clarity at all levels on the first response, the contact persons in the communication team, and the authorized spokespersons. If there is an event, which may likely to draw media attention, it is a good practice to proactively sensitize stakeholders and provide the spokespersons likely questions and answers.

Investigators are often the first point of contact by journalists. Typically, investigators are trained and supported by media consultants to manage media enquiries. Investigators could be provided with reactive statements to be provided at the first contact and then they could direct the journalist to sponsor's communication team. The designated spokespersons of sponsors could then answer the journalists on specific questions.

There are broadly few fundamental principles while managing such situations (i) to provide simple, clear, concise, factual, and consistent messages in a professional manner (ii) to reassure the stakeholders in a proactive and transparent manner (iii) to uphold the credibility and reputation of all parties to maintain trust. As there is a propensity of distortion of messages and utmost care is necessary. Often time is the essence in such delicate situations.

112. Trial of the future

Human experimentation is a serious scientific field. The clinical trial operation has evolved over the years to be more ethical and transparent. Human rights, safety, and data credibility have been the major focus areas in clinical research for several decades. Currently, the field is highly regulated and process intensive to meet the expectations. The science is constantly evolving with the changing health care delivery paradigms and greater clarity on ethical research principles.

The next area of focus is a way of trial conduct that is more inclusive and patient-friendly. There is a growing awareness in the general population about the importance of clinical trials for newer and safer therapies. Significant efforts and investments are currently underway to transform the way trials are conducted so that while taking part in a trial, subjects can pursue their normal daily lives with minimal disruption. Trials of the future, as envisaged would be less cumbersome not only for those who volunteer but also for all stakeholders. Here are few concepts in that direction.

Remote and e-informed consent (eIC): Electronic processes can supplement or replace conventional paper consent documents. Mobile technology for remote administration, biometric or security questions for identity verification, interactive interfaces with video and audio content, dynamic assessment of comprehension, and electronic signatures to register subject consent are currently workable solutions. eIC can also help in the rapid notification of updates and passive transfer of data to trial databases.

Patient centricity: The conventional approach to clinical research has been heavily tilted towards scientific hypothesis testing to meet regulatory requirements. Collaboration with communities and patient groups can make the trials friendlier by incorporating their suggestions. Disease awareness creation in the community, patient-friendly protocol, simple informed consent process, the inclusion of diverse patient population, passive data capture, use of technology, and transparent communication of results are some of the approaches to make patients the focus of clinical research.

Wearable and mobile technology: Wearable devices to measure and send body parameters using mobile technology can lower the burden on subjects and sites while enhancing data integrity. Mobile devices with interactive interfaces can support patient interviews, collect patient measured or reported data and improve compliance using auto reminders. Such devices are a major step forward to help some of the critical steps of trial conduct remotely in natural settings.

Site-less trials: Telehealth technologies and electronic interactive web platforms can be used to conduct trial activities such as recruitment, screening, informed consent, education, and data collection with participants at their home. A coordinating center can facilitate trial activities with the help of local health care professionals who can visit subjects at their home or workplace as necessary. Trial medications can be delivered to subjects at their home or workplace. Specifically equipped mobile vans can support some of the procedures such as blood sample collection or intravenous drug administration.

Dried blood spot (DBS) testing: Blood sample collection is a major reason for a site visit by subjects. In DBS, a few drops of blood drawn by finger or heel stick onto absorbent filter papers are left to soak the paper. Such dried samples placed into plastic bags with desiccants can remain stable for a long period in ambient temperature. One at the analytical laboratory, the specimen can be extracted using automated technologies for testing. Such techniques can support the concept of the site less trial conduct with minimal subject training.

Data analytics: Use of machine learning concepts is already used in risk-based monitoring. Analytics on secondary data such as electronic health records, insurance claims, prescription records, etc can help finding the right investigational sites with the right patient population. Such approaches can also help in optimization of trial designs to be in-sync with the real patients. With the wide use of IT systems in clinical trials and consequent data generation, big data analytics is expected to play a vital role to optimize processes, risk identification, and event prediction.